'I am a Woman
Phenomenally.
Phenomenal Woman,
that's me.'

MAYA ANGELOU

TO DARLING CLEMMY, BIBI & BEN

About Annie Auerbach
Annie Auerbach is a speaker, consultant, brand strategist and the co-founder of trends agency Starling, which specializes in helping brands understand cultural change in order to stay relevant. Starling's clients include Pepsico, Nike and Unilever. Annie was named a 2019 Timewise Power Founder on #timewisepower50 alongside a range of flex working trailblazers who are changing the future of work. She has worked flexibly for twenty years in many different guises—part-time, remote working, freelancing, through a portfolio career and returning to work after having her two daughters. She lives in London with her family.

Find out more about Annie and FLEX at
https://starlingstrategy.co.uk/flexthebook/

flex

Annie
Auerbach

HQ
An imprint of HarperCollinsPublishers Ltd
1 London Bridge Street
London SE1 9GF

www.harpercollins.co.uk

HarperCollins*Publishers*
1st Floor, Watermarque Building, Ringsend Road
Dublin 4, Ireland

This edition 2021

1
First published in Great Britain by
HQ, an imprint of HarperCollinsPublishers Ltd 2019

Cover design: © HarperCollins
Page design by Louise Evans

A catalogue record for this book is
available from the British Library.

ISBN: 978-0-00-840042-2

Printed and bound in the UK by CPI Group (UK) Ltd

MIX
Paper from
responsible sources
FSC™ C007454

THIS

~

IS

~

FLEX

F lex is a manifesto for living and working on your terms. It means looking at the established, rigid ways of doing things and asking: 'Is this really working for me?' If the answer to that question is 'No' then read on, because this book is for you.

When we learn how to flex we gain a superpower that allows us to challenge what is holding us back and reinvent the rules for a smarter, happier life. Because things are changing for women across the globe. We are getting married and having children later, if at all. Dual-income families have replaced the traditional template of man as breadwinner and woman as homemaker. Technology allows us to work differently and understand ourselves better.

But the old systems still persist. We're continually bashing up against inflexible structures that were built by, and for, men. We are trying to do everything, but following a rulebook we didn't write.

Cartoons of working women depict us as harassed multi-taskers with eight octopus arms, juggling food, lipstick, laptop and wine. Who actually wants to live their lives like this? Who wants to be a jittery octopus lady constantly time-pressed and on the verge of meltdown? Not me.

I've been thinking about flex for a long time. I've worked flexibly for 20 years in many different guises – part-time, remote working, through a portfolio career and freelancing. I am now 40, I run my own business and I have two daughters under 10, a husband and a small snappy dog – so I am right in the eye of the storm.

In 2016, I founded a cultural insights agency called Starling with my business partner, Adam. At Starling, we help brands understand how society is changing, so they can be more relevant. We speak to the smartest academics and the most radical thinkers. We ask 'why?'; we listen out for what's being ignored; we help our clients build better futures. And so I decided to use this approach to look at the old structures that are restricting us, and come up with shiny new solutions. Researching how women are working and living today turned out to be an awakening for me.

I have encountered a huge number of people who have found different ways to flex. These pioneers of flexible working may have initially been motivated by the need to manage childcare and responsibilities at home as well as progressing in their careers, but they are also unrecognized revolutionaries who have been chipping away at the systems that society has outgrown. They refuse to accept the status quo, they challenge handed-down wisdom and they change the game for the rest of us. Quite simply, they are phenomenal, and we need to learn from them. In each chapter, I've featured a story from one of these pioneering flexers.

I wrote this book because I'm inspired by them, and I think the image of stressed, juggling womanhood is past its sell-by date. I don't want to join the army of knackered octopus women, desperately hashtagging #wineoclock and marching under the banner of 'having it all'. I don't want to be told I have to be good at everything, all of the time. Friendship, leadership, parenting, Pilates, make-up, public speaking, cake baking, sodding tennis. It's exhausting, it's not cool and I'm over it.

More and more businesses in different sectors are recognizing the fundamental importance of creativity in their employees, whatever their role, yet we seem to be funnelling ourselves into tighter and more restrictive routines and thinking patterns. When we prioritize the wrong things – like long working hours over friendships; exams over mental agility; climbing the established career ladder over cutting our own paths – we diminish and inhibit ourselves and our possibilities.

Similarly, when we ignore our bodies' moods and cycles, going against the grain of how we feel or what we really want, then we can only really feel like we're failing, living half-lives.

Flex is a creative, rebellious, badass way to live, because it means looking at routines like the nine-to-five, and social norms like women bearing the brunt of the emotional load at home, and bending and re-shaping them. When you flex, you invent your own template, according to your own ambitions and your family's needs, often without precedent on a truly blank slate.

So to flex we need to be brave. We need to take a long look within and ask, 'How can I work to the best of my abilities at work, while being the mum or partner or friend I want to be at home?' And once we've figured out what exactly flex means for us as individuals, we have to find the confidence go out there and ask for it. Even when it goes against our current climate of pointless meetings, presenteeism, the strictures of nine-to-five and even society's expectations on us as women. And I want to show you how. The five chapters of this book ask what the concept of flex looks like through different lenses: work, yes, but also our minds, our homes, our bodies and finally our futures.

We know that the world is changing fast. Rigidity in a world of change means something is going to break, and that thing could be you. And think about it: many of the jobs we were trained for in school won't exist in a decade. The more robotic our behaviour, the more vulnerable we are to the robots taking our place. So flex has to be, for all of us, a movement built on creativity, bravery, anti-convention and innovation.

When we learn to flex, we reinvent the rules for a new future, and it's one in which we can all thrive.

'Think left and think right, and think low and think high. Oh, the Thinks you can think up if only you try.'

DR SEUSS

FLEX

~

YOUR

~

MIND

My day job is coming up with fresh thinking and new ideas for brands. I love ideas. I love the first sniff of one, the gut feeling we're onto something. The hunt for more evidence and the inevitable period of doubt and being 'lost in the forest'. The joy of getting it down on paper. I love all of it.

Flex is about inventing new answers to old problems and picking at the threads of handed-down wisdom to see what unravels. It means having a low boredom threshold for the 'same old, same old'. It makes us challenge the status quo and ask difficult questions, like: is this the way we should be living and working? Are the norms we've all bought into making us happy? This is opposite of dogma and rigidity. It is a sort of cognitive yoga; an exercise for the mind that stretches our horizons and challenges our biases. It requires bravery, leaps of faith and empathy. And, annoyingly, it's not easy . . .

Some days at work, my partner Adam and I are creative ninjas. Other days, we talk about last night's telly and what we're going to have for lunch. Creativity isn't effortless, there's no app for it, but it's vital if we are to find new and exciting ways to change the things that are restricting us. In this chapter, I'll dig into the key ingredients for creativity, so that we can unlock it in ourselves. I will look at how our environments have conspired against us to make us inflexible and I'll show how we can foster the right conditions for creativity to thrive.

Today, whether you're a coffee barista or a CEO, everyone hungers to be creative. The *New Yorker* dubs it 'Creativity Creep' saying: 'Few qualities are more sought after, few skills more envied. Everyone wants to be more creative – how else, we think, can we become fully realized people?'[1]

Part of this is because we have more time to spend on being creative. As Walter Pitkin observed back in 1932, thanks to medical breakthroughs and time-saving devices like washing machines, 'Men and women alike turn from the ancient task of *making a living* to the strange new task of *living*.' And *living* these days is a creative endeavour. Social media has fetishized visually beautiful lives. Even if we're making a packed lunch for our children, it's got to be inventive, stylish, Instagrammable.

Instagram is full of creativity quotes from smart people. 'Creativity is not a talent. It is a way of operating.' 'Creativity is intelligence having fun!' 'You can mimic a result. But not the creativity.' These all sound nice and inspiring. You can imagine the fist pumps, the head nods.

But what does creative thinking actually mean?

EVOLUTION & DAD JOKES: WHAT IS CREATIVITY?

I want to start by looking at a classic case of creativity, a leap in thinking which for ever changed the conversation for humankind: the Theory of Evolution. The fascinating thing about this idea is that it occurred to two different people, Charles Darwin and Alfred Russel Wallace, independently. For two separate thinkers to reach the same place at the same time is a real rarity.

So what did they do in order to get to their big idea? In an essay published in 1959, American sci-fi writer Isaac Asimov looked at what their creative processes had in common to try to find the key to creativity.[2]

Firstly, they travelled. Darwin took a five-year, round-the-world trip aboard HMS *Beagle* in 1831. Wallace went to the Amazon and Rio Negro river basins in 1848, and then, in 1854, to the Malay Archipelago.

Secondly, both observed unfamiliar species of plants and animals and how they varied from place to place.

Darwin famously went to the Galápagos Islands to study finches, tortoises and mockingbirds. During his travels in what is modern-day Indonesia, Wallace collected more than 100,000 insect, bird and animal specimens, which he donated to British museums.

Thirdly, both read Thomas Malthus's *An Essay on the Principle of Population*, which predicted that the human population would grow faster than its ability to feed itself. This proved to unlock the puzzle for both men. Reading about overpopulation in human beings sparked their ideas on evolution by natural selection. That's how Wallace and Darwin made their creative leap: by connecting two seemingly unconnected concepts.

Cross-connection may be the key to creativity. The *Oxford English Dictionary* definition of creativity is 'the use of imagination or original ideas to create something', but this seems like quite a stretch. Is there really such a thing as pure originality, an idea that has never been thought of before? But smashing together two existing ideas which have never been connected – that is a breakthrough. That is what makes creative friction and sparks something fresh.

Smashing together two
existing ideas which have
never been connected –
that is a breakthrough.

That is what makes
creative friction and sparks
something fresh.

As the psychologist Steven Pinker has observed, that is how jokes work. In his book *The Act of Creation*, Arthur Koestler says we laugh when one idea, or frame of reference, sits next to a second, which doesn't initially seem to make sense in the context of the first. So here's a joke: Lady Astor supposedly said to Winston Churchill, 'If you were my husband, I'd put poison in your tea.' He replied, 'If you were my wife, I'd drink it.'

Why is this funny? Well, clearly no one wants to be murdered. But when we gear-shift to suicide as a welcome escape from poor old Lady Astor, it becomes funny.

This slamming together of two unexpected frames, where the latter is surprising and causes you to reconsider the former, is called a paraprosdokian (from the Greek 'against expectation'). Paraprosdokians are what the rest of us might call 'dad jokes'. Like Stephen Colbert's: 'If I am reading this graph correctly – I'd be very surprised.' And Groucho Marx's: 'I've had a perfectly wonderful evening, but this wasn't it.'

Koestler's *The Act of Creation* looks beyond comedy to art and science. Creativity in these disciplines, he thought, is also about exploring the relationship between two unrelated ideas. He calls this 'bisociation'.

For him, creativity is the bisociation of two self-contained but incompatible frames of reference. In short, a dad joke.

IT'S HARDER THAN EVER TO BE CREATIVE TODAY

But it is not as simple as that. We've become really bad at bisociation. Creativity may be higher on the cultural agenda, and it might be a key skill for the future, but the truth is, it is now harder to be creative.

Why is this? Today, we simply don't have the bandwidth to be creative. Our technology both overwhelms and distracts us. Every 24 hours people are bombarded with the equivalent of 34 gigabytes of information – that amount would overload a laptop within a week.[3] We can't calmly absorb all this information and metabolize it into beautiful creative thought.

Digital overload is making us act like Dug, the talking dog in Pixar's movie *Up*. Every few moments, he interrupts himself mid-speech, ears pricked, nose quivering and shouts, 'SQUIRREL!' Dug is all of us, except our squirrels are tweet storms; siren calls from abandoned, half-filled online shopping carts; the jerk of the leash when we are tagged in a photo.

So we're too distracted to be creative. But even if we manage to focus, our own creativity – our ability to bisociate – is under threat from algorithms. When Amazon nudges us to buy a similar book to the one we've just clicked on, when Netflix cues up yet another film 'with a strong female lead', when social media echo chambers only feed us news that is palatable to us, we're

THE STATE OF PERMA-DISTRACTION
Gloria Mark studies digital distraction at the University of California. She has found that it takes about 23 minutes to return to the original task after an interruption. So that quick minute spent on Twitter or Facebook isn't just 60 seconds. It's 24 minutes down the drain.[4]

being pigeon-holed. We're being funnelled down a narrow path. Instead of the quirky, interesting people we imagine ourselves to be, we're becoming self-fulfilling prophecies, living in a bland monoculture. All of this amounts to a navel-gazing outlook (or in-look) which keeps us thinking in the ways we have always thought. We are stuck in a monotonous spin-cycle of our own experience, which is a profoundly uncreative place to be.

'Everyone thinks they are right all the time about everything,' innovation strategist Faris Yakob told me. 'We can't see anyone else's point of view with clarity. We assume they are idiots and racists. It's got to the point where I can't emotionally understand a position that is different from mine. I tend to like reading books about history and politics, but I'm forcing myself to read more fiction. Reading fiction helps you develop empathy and understand better where people you disagree with are coming from.'

We also bristle at any opinion that differs from our own. Ian Martin, writer on political comedy *The Thick of It*, called Twitter a 'shrieking tunnel of fuck'. In the midst of this polarized battleground it is harder than ever to find common ground, to flex our positions and move forward. Without respect for another's perspectives or empathy for their experiences, we can't make connections, bisociate and progress our thinking. Remember, the dictionary definition tells us creativity is: 'the use of imagination or original ideas to create something'. Ouch. Cultural zombies can't be creative, can they? Shrieking trolls won't open their imagination, will they? How can we escape our 'tunnel of fuck' and find the fuel for empathy and inventiveness?

STEREOTYPING + CREATIVITY

Evidence suggests that lack of empathy for others is indeed a block to creativity. A 2012 study by Tel Aviv University found that people who 'believe that racial groups have fixed underlying essences' did not do as well in creative tests as those who saw racial categories as 'arbitrary and malleable'. So those who pigeonhole racial groups have 'a habitual closed-mindedness that . . . hampers creativity', the study authors wrote.[5]

BECOMING
T-SHAPED

The creative industries are always on the hunt for what they call 'T-shaped' people. The vertical bit of the T – the I – is depth of experience in a specific subject. The horizontal bit of the T is a broader range of experience across subjects, which encompasses the capacity to peek over the top of parapets, to collaborate, to find links between different disciplines. Essentially, the horizontal bit of the T is the knack of Koestler's bisociation. So this magical T-shaped human combines the vertical skill of rigour and the horizontal skill of empathy.

But it's really hard to be T-shaped these days. The vertical is being fuelled, meaning we are being made more I-shaped by the algorithms that feed us more and more of what we already know. But the horizontal – empathy – needs our active attention. Cross-pollination requires us to break out of our echo chambers, broaden our horizons and open our hearts and minds to the new.

Travel is one way to do this. Remember both Darwin and Wallace were committed explorers. Faris Yakob and his wife Rosie are nomadic creatives who travel around the world working for their consultancy Genius Steals. Travel is very important to them. Faris told me: 'Habituation makes you blind. It turns your brain off.' Rosie says travel turns it back on again. 'There's a discomfort to being in new places,' she explains. 'It means you need to notice and be curious. The more you travel and the stranger the situations you are in, the more likely you are to expand your surface area and serendipitous things might happen.'

It's not enough to simply go on holiday. Two weeks on a sun lounger in Majorca won't cut the creative mustard. You have to do what Rosie talked about: notice things, be curious, talk to people, figure out new ways of doing things.

Not all of us can afford the luxury of travelling in order to boost creativity, of course. But many of us can at the very least get out of the workplace and go for a walk. Research from Creative Equals, an organization that champions diversity in the creative industries, shows that just 9 per cent of people have their best ideas in the office. Fans of the walking meeting include Arianna Huffington, Mark Zuckerberg and Barack Obama.

The first reason to go for a walk is that we need to move more. We're living in sedentary times, sitting on average, for 9.3 hours per day, longer than we are sleeping.[6] The second reason is to boost our creativity. Researchers at Stanford University asked people to think up new uses for common objects while sitting at a desk or walking. Over three-quarters came up with more ideas while walking than sitting.[7]

At Starling, Adam and I walk to client meetings rather than taking the Tube. It means we leave in good time and don't rush. We use the journey to discuss the meeting ahead, or just chat. Some of our best ideas and conversations happen on walks – a time which otherwise would be a deadzone of getting from A to B.

Walking is second nature. It doesn't require concentration. It allows the mind to wander. The state of the wandering mind has been shown to be fertile for creative ideas and flashes of insight. When we don't try hard to have an idea – sod's law – it comes to us.

HOW TO BE
T-SHAPED

~

1. Travel. And if you can't travel, be open to new influences wherever they might be – notice things, be curious, ask why. Take a new route to work or school. This will force you to see things slightly differently and confront you with new inputs.

2. Go for a walk on your own, and let ideas sneak up on you. Or with someone else and talk them through.

3. Take a photo each day. This will nudge you to observe, to look harder at everyday things you may otherwise ignore and find new perspectives.

4. Break your echo chamber. I have scrutinized who I follow on Twitter and my aim now is to follow diverse, challenging voices and avoid the loud, obvious ones.

5. Be empathetic. Try to think flexibly and openly about ideas that feel odd and jarring to you.

6. Clash these ideas together, make connections, join dots. Tell dad jokes.

7. Read books. Fiction, non-fiction, anything. Just keep reading.

8. And read things you wouldn't automatically choose. Take inspiration from Stack. Stack is a subscription service that delivers a different specialist magazine each month, on anything from art to tennis.

9. Be OK with having creative droughts. Don't panic. When this happens, see points 2 and 7.

10. Take the pressure off yourself, be in the moment, don't force it. That's when the magic will happen.

PINNY GRYLLS' FLEX STORY

*Pinny Grylls is a documentary filmmaker
and children's author*

My worst ideas come from sitting on the internet and researching things. You are at a computer, your eyeballs are staring at the screen, there's a digital wall between you and a real story, which has already been mediated several times. I want to get to a new story, a new perspective, not one already told by someone else.

You need to get off your arse and actually physically meet people. Ordinary day-to-day conversations and events can be doors into new ideas and films. An example of this: I was buying a second-hand car and had to pick it up from Stoke-on-Trent. It was going to be a boring task – collecting the car, signing documents and whatnot. But I was sitting in this guy's living room, and he told me he works as a hypnotist, specializing in doing past-life regression with traumatized people who work in the fire service. These people had ordinary lives, they were not novelists or professional creatives. Yet, under his care, they pop into another realm and become someone else. They tell stories of being a nineteenth-century farmer committing a murder, or a priest in Tibet. I was inspired to make a film about it and it became a Channel 4 documentary.

I try not to impose a story on the world. The way I work is a collaboration between me and the person who wants their story to be told, who wants it to be witnessed. That's why you need to meet people, to get the magic, the intimacy. You don't get it from a screen. You have to be with them physically.

My tip is to give yourself permission not to work. Go on a road trip to buy that second-hand car. It may be a more interesting day than you thought. Don't force yourself to sit at a screen and come up with ideas. Do the washing up. Read a story to your kid. Do ordinary things, and your brain will go somewhere else. Take pressure off those moments and let 'being' in your life be enough. When you take pressure off, that's when you find things.

I was diagnosed with a two-centimetre wide benign brain tumour which was right between my eyes. I had radiation therapy and they had to scan it every six months. We took time off work and school and went on a family campervan road trip around Europe. We thought, 'We don't know what the future is, so we want do this now.' Recently, I had a scan to see whether the radiation had worked. If it hadn't, I needed a dangerous operation to remove it. It had shrunk by 25 per cent, I was given the all-clear and it was like being given my life back.

Until that point, I didn't realize I had been in stasis, not being able to plan anything. But ironically, this had allowed me to be more in the moment and to live! We cram so much into our days; we pressure ourselves. We're a culture that is geared up for quantifiable achievement and status. It's hard to get out of that way of thinking. We need to be patient, to give ourselves permission to dream and not fill every moment of downtime. We need to 'be' and believe it doesn't matter if nothing creative comes out of it. It's enough being alive. That is the ultimate creative act.

LIBERTY & RESTRAINT

It's tempting to see creativity as relying on complete freedom and expansiveness. Many have found that the opposite is true. Creativity can thrive when there are restrictions and barriers in place. It is these roadblocks which can force breakthroughs. David Ogilvy, the advertising guru known as the original Mad Man, once said, 'Give me the freedom of a tight brief'. What did he mean by this?

Limits give you clarity, focus and purpose. They also give you a feeling of safety, and safety gives you the confidence to explore.

BEAUTIFUL CONSTRAINTS

Adam Morgan and Mark Barden's book, *A Beautiful Constraint: How to Transform Your Limitations into Advantages*, refers to a study of children's playground habits. In a playground in a wide open field where they could run anywhere, children tended to stay in the middle. When faced with complete freedom, it feels more reassuring to be near the other kids, to keep the status quo. However, if you build a fence around the field, children will explore right to the edge and use the whole space. Ironically, in a contained, safe space, you can roam free.

So think about fences for your creativity. Put in some 'beautiful constraints' and you might push yourself beyond the status quo. When Olivia Laing wrote her novel *Crudo*, her 'fences' were that she would write every day and she wasn't allowed to go back and edit. She finished it in seven weeks. She said: 'Because there was no intention or plan, I wasn't self-conscious and I wasn't worried about trying to get perfect sentences, it was just smashing them down as fast as I could.'

If you are a procrastinator, your 'fence' could be a strict time limit on the task ahead. If you are the sort of person who makes long lists about what you need to get done, reduce them to one bullet point. This is your creative objective for the day.

Constraints also make you work harder to be creative and push you to excel. Jerry Seinfeld bans himself from jokes containing sex or swearing – it's just too easy to get a laugh. These limits raised his game and upped his comic creativity. He says: 'A person who can defend themselves with a gun is just not very interesting. But a person who defends themselves through aikido or tai chi? Very interesting.'[8] He treats his stand-up sessions as scientific experiments, analysing the type and length of laugh he gets for each joke and using that analysis to shave off a word, honing his routine until it is pitch perfect. For him, the creativity lies in what's left out.

If you have creative paralysis, write a list of everything this is NOT. So if, say, you are planning a hen party for a friend, write down everything she would hate first of all. These are your guardrails – and you can create freely within them.

Think about fences
for your creativity...
and you might push
yourself beyond
the status quo.

Rules can give you freedom from interruption. We've seen how insidious digital distraction can be today, sapping much more real time than the actual diversion took. The writer Zadie Smith has a zero tolerance policy towards social media and doesn't connect to the internet during her writing time, leaving any fact checking until she has finished writing for the day. 'If I could control myself online, if I wasn't going to go down a Beyoncé Google hole for four and a half hours, this wouldn't be a problem. But that is exactly what I'll do,' she says.

Experiment with using airplane mode on your phone, and setting strict times of the day (at the beginning and the end) in which to deal with emails. Use apps like Freedom and Self Control which allow you to block your own access to websites, apps or the entire internet to stop wasting time online. Use time before bed to read, rather than being on your phone – stretch your empathy muscles.

Creativity also requires chutzpah. Chutzpah is a Yiddish word that refers to self-confidence or bravery. Clashing disciplines, making the connections, bisociation: none of this can be done by someone suffering from self-doubt. You needed swagger to say the Earth was round when everyone thought it was flat. You need guts to walk away from accepted wisdom. 'The difficulty lies not so much in developing new ideas,' said John Maynard Keynes, 'as in escaping from old ones.'

CHANNEL YOUR CHUTZPAH

Escaping the 'old ones' can be hard because they've been handed down to us as gospel. Our parents might have even embedded these ideas in our bedtime stories. And moving away from them makes a statement that you do not need their (or society's) approval any more.

We can all do this, but what gets in the way is the belief that creativity only lies in the hands of very few select people. The notion that true creatives are artists, misfits at the edges of society or geniuses who are 'ahead of their time' is a barrier to creativity. It lets you say: 'Creativity lives in others, but not in me.' It stops you being brave and robs you of your chutzpah.

One of the most generous and powerful speeches on this comes from the Australian comedian Hannah Gadsby. In her game-changing performance 'Nanette', she takes a swipe at the 'great men of art' school of thought, which characterizes people like Van Gogh and Picasso as lone, eccentric geniuses.

Gadsby says: 'People believe that Van Gogh was just this misunderstood genius, born ahead of his time. What a load of shit. Nobody is born ahead of their time! It's impossible . . . Artists don't invent zeitgeists, they respond to them . . . [Van Gogh] was not ahead of his time. He was a post-Impressionist painter painting at the peak of post-Impressionism.'

We're all products of our time. We all swim in the cultural soup. Our creativity comes from how we respond to it. Bravery, daring, escaping the old ideas – we can have them all. We just need the chutzpah to do so.

We all swim in
the cultural soup.
Our creativity comes
from how we
respond to it.

HOW TO CHANNEL
YOUR CHUTZPAH

~

1. Notice the moments when you have been brave in
   the past. When you owned up to a mistake. Or you
   called out an injustice. Why did you do it? How
   did you feel? If you recognize and cherish those
   moments, you can summon them again when you
   are in need of chutzpah.

2. Don't feel self-conscious and let it inhibit your ideas.
   No one is thinking about you. That sounds a bit sad,
   but it's actually liberating. No one is thinking of
   you! They are too busy thinking about themselves.
   Remember Coco Chanel's words: 'I don't care what
   you think about me. I don't think about you at all.'

3. Work out who diminishes your bravery. Who is your Achilles heel? Who do you always feel sheepish or inhibited around? These people are drains. Instead, try to hang around people who boost your mojo.

4. Done is better than perfect. Obsessing about perfection is navel-gazing and paralyzing. Get it done, get it out, get on with life.

5. If all else fails channel Dolly Parton. She said: 'Find out who you are. And do it on purpose.'

Then dare, shed the old assumptions – and create.

SUMMARY

Modern life is conspiring to make us into cultural zombies. Creativity is scarcer and more urgent than ever. In order to flex we need to interrogate what we really want, and what we need to change to get it – and to do this we must have the space to think creatively. Creativity is a muscle that needs exercising – think of it as cognitive yoga – in order to dodge the algorithmic monoculture that wants to swallow us up.

So when an idea hits you, let it run. Comedian Dave Chappelle says that for him, creativity involves letting go. 'If I have an idea, it's the driver. The idea says, "Get in the car," and I'm like, "Where am I going?" The idea says, "I don't know. Don't worry about it. I'm driving." Sometimes I'm shotgun, sometimes I'm in the fucking trunk. The idea takes you where it wants to go.' [9]

Let your ideas take you where they want to go. Swim in the cultural soup, read books, react to what's out there. Listen to people, meet them face to face, empathize with them, look them in the eye and connect with them. Don't try and be ahead of your time; be of your time and say something different about it.

But, most importantly, trust in yourself, be brave and nourish your own chutzpah. Creativity doesn't live in the hands of lone geniuses. It lives in us all.

'Working nine to five,
what a way to make a living.
Barely getting by, it's all taking
and no giving.

They just use your mind,
and they never give you credit.
It's enough to drive you crazy
if you let it.'

DOLLY PARTON

FLEX

~

YOUR

~

WORK

was a director at a global research agency. Six months earlier I'd given birth to my second daughter. I had come back to work after maternity leave and negotiated a part-time, three-day-a-week contract. I'd achieved the holy grail: flexibility. I could look after my baby and three-year-old whilst holding down the job I loved. I should have been triumphant, clicking my heels together as I trotted off into the sunset, swinging a laptop case in one hand and a nappy bag in the other, the clichéd stock image of a working woman.

But, no. It was a disaster. It was one of the most pressurized and stressful periods of my life, peppered with moments when I felt I was failing. Here are some examples:

~ When I left work bang on time and felt my colleagues' raised eyebrows and disapproval haunt me as I galloped to the Tube station.

~ When I arrived sweating, frazzled and tense to take over from the nanny for the battleground of a toddler bathtime.

~ When I sat on the loo seat and mindlessly chugged a ten-minute Instagram fix.

~ When I worked more, unpaid, than my three
   allotted days, answering emails on days off and
   writing reports after I put my daughter to bed.

~ When I frantically tapped out a work email at the
   edge of the sandpit, whilst my daughter got into
   fist-fights over buckets and spades.

I remember a poignant news story during this period.
The number of playground accidents was apparently
on the rise. Kids were falling off climbing frames, being
flattened by swings and jettisoned from seesaws. I linked
it with the hordes of distracted mums like me, squinting
over iPhones on benches at the edges of the playground,
trying to reply to incessant requests from colleagues on
their days off. My failed flexibility would land my kid in
hospital, I was sure of it.

And even if it didn't, I still felt guilty that those precious
two days with my daughter were so un-fun. I was un-
fun. I was exhausted, constantly multi-tasking, never
focused on the present, mind swivelling to the next task.
I was like one of those terrible people at parties who
keep looking over your shoulder in case there's a sexier
guest – except I was doing that to my own daughter.

And the sexy guest was a boring email about a work meeting. And yet all the time, throughout this period, I felt grateful. Grateful to my bosses for giving me the chance to feel like I was failing in every respect.

I know. Get the violins out. All of this constitutes a 'First-World problem'. Things were largely OK, and I'm sure my story is no different to any other working parent's. But clearly, flexibility, as I had it, was a shitshow.

I wanted to understand why it was such a fiasco when I tried to flex my working hours around parenthood. And why are we all so wedded to the nine-to-five, five days a week?

I found, as I will show in this chapter, that it's not enough to simply convince your employers to agree to flexibility, as I had done. This is just the beginning. The flexible arrangement actually needs to work, too. And that requires new ways of thinking from both the employer and the employee.

This chapter will look at our modern relationship with time and understand why the nine-to-five (or longer) has become the norm. I will explain what is

currently broken within work culture today – the
pressures and rigidity that are making people ill, sad
and overwhelmed. I will examine the concept of flexible
working that seeks to address work and life, without
feeling that we are failing at both. And I will give tips
on how to achieve flexible working that works, for
everyone. The story begins – let's face it, it often does –
in sixteenth-century Italy.

GALILEO, COFFEE BREAKS & SYNCHRONIZED TIME

Galileo Galilei, a 19-year-old student at the University
of Pisa, is attending mass at the Duomo di Pisa. The
year is 1583. Let's imagine he is bored and his mind is
wandering. He's staring at the ceiling when he notices
a lamp swinging on a long metal chain. As Stephen
Johnson explains in *How We Got to Now*, 'No matter
how long the arc, the lamp seems to take the same
amount of time to swing back and forth.' Galileo can't
test this out by timing it on his watch. Watches don't

exist yet, and nor do particularly reliable clocks. So Galileo measures the swing of the lamp against his own pulse. And the idea for a pendulum clock is born.

The pendulum clock changed our relationship with time. Back in the sixteenth century, there were no accurate clocks, but, never having had them, no one really missed them. People weren't racing for trains, rushing home to watch the football or dialling into another unnecessary conference call at 1.45 p.m. Everyone was on their own, meandering, unaligned schedule.

Precise synchronized time, as we think of it now, is a modern concept, born out of the Industrial Revolution. Factory work, clocking in and out, taking tea and lunch breaks when instructed to by the boss – all of this built to a sense of co-ordinated time, with strict divisions between work and leisure. When Welsh social reformer Robert Owen fought for an eight-hour working day in 1817, demanding, 'Eight hours labour, eight hours recreation, eight hours rest', these rhythms became synchronized habits and the modern nine-to-five was born.

That suited an industrial economy. But today, across the world, we are moving from a manufacturing-based economy to a service-based economy. Service-based economies are dominated by tourism, social work, creative industries, retail and media, amongst others. Of course, there are some jobs where flexibility is harder to manage – doctors, police officers, call-centre workers who need to cover specific hours. But many of us who sit at desks should have more control of our time.

We need to get the job done, but surely when, where and how is up to us. Yet the hangover of fixed, long hours prevails.

Why is this?

Dale Southerton, professor of sociology of consumption at the University of Bristol, is an expert on time usage. He told me that throughout society there are 'traces and resonances of past temporal rhythms'. Which is why we automatically fancy a cup of tea and a biscuit at 11 a.m., almost as if the factory morning break is imprinted on our collective memories.

Despite having more control over our time in a service-based economy, we slip into the habits and timings of previous generations. Southerton talked of the etymology of the word 'routine'. It comes from the French 'route', or road. He used the metaphor of a muddy track through a field. Even though we can walk through the field in any direction, we tend to follow the track that previous walkers have left. Throughout society, groups and businesses follow paths, rhythms and routines which previous generations have established. There's a safety to it: you won't fall down a hole or get lost and you'll avoid hidden snakes in the grass.

But the safety is deceptive. Doing what we've always done and keeping to outmoded timings and rhythms is actually dangerous, both to our own health and the health of businesses. Presenteeism – being present at your place of work for more hours than required – and burn-out – exhaustion through overwork – are two of the biggest issues in the modern workplace.

THE OPPOSITE OF FLEX: BURNT-OUT BUMS ON SEATS

Today, we're slaves to presenteeism. Being there in body if not in spirit. Long working hours. Working while sick.

The big irony about bums on seats is that these long-suffering bums are proving to be deeply unproductive bums. Working longer hours doesn't always translate into more productivity. Europe is facing a productivity crisis. Productivity in the UK is particularly woeful. The UK's labour productivity, usually measured as the value of goods and services produced for each hour worked, is near the bottom of the G7 league table.

The average French worker produces more by the end of Thursday than their UK equivalent does in a full week. (And that's with the French taking a long lunch and a *cinq à sept* visit to their lover – just kidding). However, Japan – home of the salaryman, crazy long hours and *Karōshi* (translation: death by overwork) – is even less productive than the UK![10]

A story about this. A Japanese friend, who is a very talented graphic designer, while working for a media firm in Tokyo, once didn't leave his office for two weeks. Two weeks! He popped to the shops to buy some pants, a toothbrush and some new shirts. But he ate, slept and worked in the office for a fortnight. All of his team did. It was expected of them as they had to meet a deadline and anyone going home would have been seen as uncommitted, a shirker. By the end of it, they were all zombies, delirious with overwork.

Clearly being present doesn't mean being productive.

~~~~~~~~~~~~~~~~~~~~~~~~~~~~~~~~~~~~~~~

PRESENT BUT NOT CORRECT

Eighty-six per cent of respondents to a 2018 UK survey said that they had seen presenteeism in their organization, up from 26 per cent in 2010.[11] This devotion to bums on seats is costing us dearly: people turning up to work while sick alone leads to a lost productivity cost of just over £4,000 per person each year on average, according to Nottingham Business School research.[12]

And yet leaving work still doesn't mean we relax. Leavism, where people are using holiday time to work, is on the up.[13] Never mind answering emails in the playground, some of us are waking up during the night to do so. One in three Britons is so stressed at work they have checked their emails in the middle of the night.[14]

Working nine-to-five (and more) is no longer fit for purpose. Unchecked, we're sleepwalking into a global mental health crisis. The Trade Union Congress found that stress brought on by long working hours and lack of job security is the top health and safety concern in workplaces. Our existing work culture in the UK is making us sick. And in Japan, it's actually killing us.

THE CALL FOR FLEX

This is where flexibility comes in. The Equality and Human Rights Commission has issued a call to action: 'We need to overhaul our culture and make flexible working the norm.'

People desperately want to work flexibly.

It's easy to assume that it's women, and in particular mums, who crave flex; to be with their children, run the home or care for their elderly relatives. And yes, it is true that mothers have been at the coalface of pushing for flexibility. But for too long it's been ghettoized, labelled a 'mum thing', a women's issue which needs to be solved by women. It's not just mums that want flexibility. Young people, old people, men and women, they all want it, too.

THE FLEX GAP

There's a gap between the desire to flex, and the availability of flexible work. US consultancy Werk found 96 per cent of the workforce needs some form of flexibility, yet only 47 per cent have access to a range of flexible options.[15] In the UK, *Marketing Week* found that 87 per cent of marketeers want flexibility, yet only 34.2 per cent have used flexible working in the last year.[16]

For young people, a good job is a flexible job. They don't envy their burnt-out bosses who never see their families. They value having control over when and how they work. Flex even trumps pay for them. A higher salary won't necessarily guarantee loyalty, but flexibility (along with diversity and inclusion) will often inspire commitment from young talent today. This might be because they want a portfolio career, and to make money from different talents on different days of the week. Or they might want to do charity work alongside their main job. They may be grafters who work into the night in the hope that their side-hustle becomes their main one. They may simply be looking for variety.

For too long it's been
ghettoized, labelled a
'mum thing', a women's
issue which needs to be
solved by women

And those a bit older, the sandwich generation who look after both elderly parents and their own children, want flexibility, too. In the US, 61 per cent of those who provide care for an older adult are also balancing jobs.[17] They need to be able to take their parents to the odd doctor's appointment in the middle of the day. Or they need to be with them at the start and end of the day, to take over from carers.

Flexibility is crucial to keeping these people – grown-up sons and daughters who care for their parents – in the workforce.

～～～～～～～～～～～～～～～～～～～～～～～～～

THE HEALTH BENEFITS OF FLEX

A review of ten studies carried out by researchers at Durham University shows mental health, blood pressure and sleep patterns were better among people who could determine their own working hours.

So all of these diverse groups can benefit practically, physically and emotionally from flexible working. But this is not just about parents, carers and younger people. Any one of us can also benefit creatively. The staff at 21212, a Michelin-starred restaurant in Edinburgh, are trialling a four-day week (without reducing their salaries) in order to boost the creative flair of the team. They believe the day off will give them the space to find fresh inspiration to bring back to work.

This idea of the four-day work week has been getting more attention recently. Whether the fifth day is spent taking the time for yourself, your hobby, or your family, it is a way of finding space for inputs instead of continual outputs. This can only improve our energy and creativity.

CAN YOU BE
MORE FLEXIBLE?

Flexible working in the broadest sense is a work practice that gives employees flexibility on how long, where and when they work. But what form of it is right for you?

All employees – not just parents and carers – have the legal right to ask for flexible working if they have been in the job for a set period of time. This varies around the world. In the UK it's 26 weeks. You should put your request in writing, date it, explain it is a statutory request and describe what you would like, when you would like it to start and how that will alter your existing arrangement. You can only make one request in any 12-month period. Your employer must consider your request seriously, but they can reject it if they believe quality, performance or standards will suffer or if additional costs are prohibitive. For a full list of reasons why employers might refuse a request, and helpful advice on the process, have a look at the Citizens Advice website.

AMELIA TORODE'S FLEX STORY

Amelia Torode is the founder of
The Fawnbrake Collective

I'd spent 20 years in London and New York working for incredible companies like Ogilvy, TBWA and WPP. As I grew more senior, my role shifted to management and developing strategies for agencies to pursue 'digital transformation'. I came to a point where I realized that I just didn't believe that 'digital transformation' of twentieth-century structures was possible.

I had a lot of time to think about this when I took time out of work to care for my mum who was battling cancer. By the end, she was really sick and it hurt her to talk, so often we just sat together as she dozed. I thought about the professional world of advertising and branding that I had stepped out of and the frustrations that I'd had about my life. When you are with someone you love, who does not have much time left, you start to think about how you spend your time, and I questioned how wisely I was spending mine. There's a wonderful Martin Luther King quote in which he talks about 'the fierce urgency of now'. I started to feel that urgency very deeply.

I launched The Fawnbrake Collective towards the end of 2017. It's a light-touch collective of entrepreneurial small businesses and independent consultants and creatives, brought together through shared values and ambitions and a belief that we solve and create better together – collaboratively, collectively – than isolated and alone. There are hundreds of Fawnbrakers, but only two full-time employees, myself and Sera Miller, my co-founder. We have a strong element of social enterprise, with pro-bono work for charities/not-for-profits woven throughout the commercial model and a commitment to genuine diversity and practical flexibility.

We wanted to get rid of as many structures that we felt were getting in the way of doing the work: so no HQ, no email, no hierarchy and no bureaucracy. When it came to thinking about talent, we believe it's not about 'owning' the people who work for you, but you need to access the best talent. Too much time is spent on professional presenteeism rather than trusting people to work the way that works best for them, so we believe in impact, not hours.

My new working life is time spent smarter. I choose the projects I want to work on, I curate the teams and I lead through example. I drop the kids at school, I have started swimming in our local lido regularly and run daily – things I could never seem to manage to do before. It's not perfect and I don't consider myself a role model, but I am trying to build something new and smarter to live the life that makes me feel challenged, engaged and balanced.

Here are some different types of flexible working you could think about:

1. **Job sharing:** two people share the work and pay of a single full-time job.

2. **Flexi-hours:** an employee works a set amount of core hours from the office, for example, 10–3 p.m. in order to do the school run, and works the remainder of their hours in their own time (for example, after 7 p.m.).

3. **Location-flex:** an employee can work at remote locations either all of the time or some of the time.

4. **One-off flex:** a worker can adapt to unforeseen circumstances (a school concert, a sick mum, even a must-see art exhibition) without being penalized, and make up those hours later.

5. **Flexi-timetabling:** people create their own working timetable which suits their own needs – for example, night owls could work an 11 a.m.–7 p.m. day, or those with awkward commutes could work 7 a.m.– 3 p.m. to miss rush hour.

6. **Flex-banking:** you work a four-day week but get paid for a 4.5-day week and that 0.5 is banked. When the business needs you for an extended period they can give you notice, book you in and cash in the banked time.

7. **Term-time flex:** full-time work during term-time and no work in the holidays.

8. **Compressed hours:** working the equivalent of full-time hours but squashed into fewer days.

9. **Annualized hours:** working a certain number of hours over the year with flexibility about when you work. You could work regular 'core hours' and work the rest of your hours flexibly or when there's extra demand at work.

10. **Phased retirement:** older workers can reduce their hours gradually and work part-time before transitioning to full-time retirement.

Well, flexibility sounds fantastic for the workers, but is it actually beneficial for companies and organisations too?

In short, yes it is.

It is great for the culture of a business. A rising tide of evidence shows flexible working practices breed a culture of motivation, engagement and productivity.[18] Employees with flexibility are more likely to feel their ideas are valued and to believe they work in an environment that fosters diverse points of view.[19]

And the good vibes aren't just felt internally. It's great for an employer brand. Employees with access to flexibility are more willing to recommend their workplace to others than those without.

Flexible working can also help with retention. HR departments fear existing mid-level talent will leave if they don't offer flexibility. Replacing talent is expensive and flex is a reason for people to stay.

Allowing people to work from home cuts costs too: fewer people in the office simultaneously means reduced rent and running costs. It can also impact productivity and profit. At China's biggest travel agency, Ctrip, employees who were 'location independent' a few days per week were shown to be more productive than their colleagues who worked exclusively in the office, and resignations amongst this group fell by 50 per cent.

And the results showed in the bottom line: the business made about $2,000 more profit per person at home.[20]

AVOIDING
THE SHITSHOW, OR
MAKING FLEX WORK

Given these clear benefits for both workers and companies, how can we avoid the mess I made of it and get flexibility to work?

At Starling, the cultural insight agency I co-founded in 2016, we interview world experts to help us understand cultural change. One such interview was with Cindy Gallop, sex tech entrepreneur, founder of MakeLoveNotPorn and self-described lover of 'blowing shit up'. Gallop said something which made me stop and think: 'Here's a guaranteed formula for business success. Seek out and recruit the very best talent. Give that talent an inspiring and compelling vision of what you want to achieve. Then stand back. Let them work in any ways they see fit. Demonstrate how much you value and trust them. Give them a high trust working environment.'

Those words: 'Let them work in any ways they see fit. Trust them,' echoed in my head.

And I realized that, until Starling, I had never worked in a high-trust business culture. One in which I have been trusted to do my job in the way that best made sense to me, without judgement, without fearing it would hinder my chances of progression. And it struck me that without a high-trust culture, it would be near impossible for flexibility to work.

The biggest worry people have about working flexibly is that they will be perceived to be less dedicated. One of my friends told me about a recent job interview. She explained to her potential employer she would like to work one day from home – she lived a 90-minute commute away – so she could pick up the kids from school, and work extra during the time she would save on the commute. They turned her down saying it didn't sound like she was committed to the job.

There is a stigma attached to asking for flexibility. Studies show that many who ask for flex worry they will be penalized as a result – for example, given wage penalties, lower performance evaluations and fewer promotions. According to a 2016 survey, men don't take extended parental leave because they fear it will jeopardize their position at work.[21] These are all worries about 'flexism' – discrimination against flexible workers.

Without a high-trust
culture, it would be near
impossible for flexibility
to work.

I had the sense that when I asked for flexibility, I slipped into a slower track at work. The perception of my seniority and experience seemed to ebb away. It didn't feel like I was in the frame for promotion. Part-time working somehow shrouded me with an air of demotion.

People feel stigmatized for asking for flex. But perhaps with good reason, because some employers believe that flexible workers *will* skive off, play the system and be less productive.

This all shows that there is a deep trust crisis around flexible working. When leaders don't have faith that their workers will keep to their side of the bargain, they don't believe in them. They don't think the flexible working arrangement will succeed and they hand down their suspicions to the rest of the business. The upshot is low trust permeates the whole organization. This is partly to do with the embedded doctrine that a good worker works long hours (wrong on so many levels, as we've seen).

The problem is flexible working isn't 'sexy'. Stories of successful and productive flexible working need to be told loudly and proudly around the organization. People who are brilliant at what they do, and who are flexing with elegance and excellence, need to become famous at work. This will give managers the confidence to not only say yes to requests, but also really believe in them. And it will give workers who need or want flexibility the reassurance they won't be nudged onto the slow track.

There are other ways in which businesses are actively trying to make flex work. CEO of Pepsi Australia and New Zealand Robbert Rietbroek leads by example. 'Leave loudly,' he says. 'If I occasionally go at 4 p.m. to pick up my daughters, I will make sure I tell the people around me, "I'm going to pick up my children." Because if it's OK for the boss, then it's OK for middle management and new hires.'

Leaving loudly is a sign that the business respects parenthood, rather than asking its people to leave their parenthood at the door. Too often working fathers and mothers are made to apologize for the fact they are parents. They are seen as the ones who leave early, the flaky ones, the uncommitted.

YOU'VE GOT MAIL

Another sign that a business is trying to make flex work, is its attitude to email. When businesses think intentionally about email, and have policies which protect their workers from the onslaught of emails out of working hours and on the weekends, it's a signal they are thinking progressively about flexible working too. French politician Benoît Hamon speaks emphatically about the curse of connectivity for the modern worker: 'Employees physically leave the office, but they do not leave their work. They remain attached by a kind of electronic leash – like a dog. The texts, the messages, the emails – they colonize the life of the individual to the point where he or she eventually breaks down.'[22] In France, businesses with more than 50 employees are required by law to guarantee workers the 'right to disconnect' from technology after they leave the office.

In Germany, Volkswagen has blocked its servers from sending or receiving emails from smartphones between 6:15 p.m. and 7 a.m. on weekdays and weekends.

If companies put in place, and respect, boundaries about email usage and make clear what expectations are in terms of replying on days off, flex has a better chance of working. If they educate the team *around* the flexible worker to buy into these boundaries, for example ensuring they don't bombard them with emails on their days off or arrange important face-to-face meetings when they are working remotely, the system will work all the better for everyone.

Annie Crombie, a friend and brilliant CEO in the not-for-profit sector working a four-day week, talks about this. 'Most of my madness of working weekends, evenings and being on my Blackberry in the playground on my day off, stems from worrying what people think of my competence. There are days when I feel kick-arse and full of self-worth and these are the days I put my Blackberry away and push the swing with both hands.'

It astounds me she would feel inadequate given her level of experience and awesomeness (it also astounds me that she still has a Blackberry). But the lesson is clear. Believe in yourself, obey your own boundaries and push the swing with both hands.

We need to flip the idea that parenthood somehow undermines competence. Senior staff, both men and women, should set an example by taking up extended parental leave, talking about their children in the workplace and encouraging others to take up flexibility. This sends a positive message to everyone in the organization, and makes parenting a super-power in the workplace.

Parents are patient negotiators, nurturers of creativity, they are tolerant, they are resilient, they have empathy. They've developed these incredible skills outside of work, which can be transferred into the workplace. Parents are the undiscovered rockstars: in a business world beset with uncertainty, we desperately need people with experience and empathy who can get shit done. As my friend says: 'After all, who's more efficient than someone maintaining three projects and a couple of kids every day?'

But the most important sign that flexible working will actually work, is if you're working in a high-trust environment. Some pioneering companies are leading the way. One of the ways companies like Netflix and LinkedIn demonstrate their trust in their workers is to offer unlimited paid time off. As long as employees' work is done, and their boss approves, they can take as much paid holiday as they want. Netflix explains: 'It's part of our freedom and responsibility culture that we trust employees to balance doing a great job with having a balanced life.'

Businesses *can* change their ways and their systems to make flexibility work – and it shouldn't all be down to the employee. However, I've spoken to a range of business leaders, heads of HR, and CEOs and I've listened to their fears around flex. Overleaf are my tips on how to ask for flexible work and what you can do to make it work once you have it.

We need to flip the
idea that parenthood
somehow undermines
competence.

HOW TO ASK FOR
FLEX & MAKE IT WORK

~

1. **Frame your request for flexible working in terms of what it will bring to the business.** This might be the injection of ideas and influences from outside that you will bring back. It might be the contacts you make, the skills you will develop, the emotional energy that you will replenish. Banish the fear that you'll skive. (And please don't skive. It breaks the trust and ruins things for the rest of us.)

2. **Show your commitment to the business.** Explain how this longer-term arrangement will work better with your life and needs and therefore will actually make you *more* committed to your job. Banish the fear that flexibility is one foot out of the door.

3. **Remain contactable.** If you want to work remotely a few days a week, explain how contactable you can be and use tools that keep you connected (Google hangouts for meetings, Google docs for shared document writing). Slack, a private space for workplace team messaging and sharing, is a

great tool to make you feel part of a team even if you are not in the office. It's good for both sharing knowledge and also the little stuff like the funny cat gifs. It's important that flex doesn't isolate you; even though you don't have the same rhythms as the rest of the team, you still need to feel like you belong.

4. **If you are working fewer days or hours, be explicit with your colleagues when you are working and when you are not.** Set up a clear out-of-office email with the times you will answer emails and the times you are out of contact. And then obey your own rules. That bears repeating – obey your own rules! If you set a precedent of replying to emails on your days off, you'll unleash the genie. You need to feel confident in your own abilities and be strong in order to resist any diligent urge you have to get back to people immediately.

SUMMARY

A workforce sitting for long hours every day in the office is not a team of people doing their best work: they are more likely to be stressed and burnt out, feeling under-appreciated, unable to care in the way they want to for the people they love, and prepared to leave in a second if they could find a job which offers them the flex they crave.

The conversation about flexible working needs to change. There's a parallel to be made with the issue of diversity in the workplace. The language has changed towards 'inclusion' – it's not enough to be diverse, although that is a start. We need to be truly inclusive, and leave the old boys' club and the 'in jokes' behind. To make a diverse workforce feel genuinely included we know we need to create the right conditions so they can thrive and do their best work.

Exactly the same shift needs to happen around flexible working. There needs to be a revolution within working culture to acknowledge the failings of rigid and long hours, address 'flexism' and actually allow for the *inclusion* of flexible workers. The result will show that flex isn't token, isn't a shitshow and actually works.

And it needs to work for everyone, not just mums. We need flexibility to work for older people, for men, for young people entering the workforce and, of course, for the businesses themselves.

This is why I care about flex so deeply. It is for anyone who has a life and a passion outside of work. Sons and daughters who need to be there for elderly parents. Talented people who believe in portfolio careers. Those that simply want to spend a little more time on something outside the four walls of their job. Flex is for any of us. And any of us should be able to make it work.

'Mother told me a couple of years ago, "Sweetheart, settle down and marry a rich man." I said, "Mom, I am a rich man."'

CHER

FLEX

~

YOUR

~

HOME

'm standing on a stage in a very beige auditorium, about to give a speech to an audience of clients who are all staring at their phones. They seem drugged by the venue's wilting pastries and bad coffee. I'm taking a breath. My heels are too high, my mouth is dry. I have my Powerpoint slides projected on a screen behind me, the clicker is in my hand. I'm going to blow their minds with my talk on consumer segmentation. This stuff is gold. Pie charts. Snazzy fonts. I'm totally ready.

But my mind is elsewhere.

Today is my daughter's first day at school. That morning she looked so solemn in her green uniform and shiny shoes, swamped by her giant blazer. She stood on the front doorstep of our home and we took a photo, but her smile was a bit wobbly. The rest of me may be in a conference centre, but my heart is with her. I check my watch, it must be morning break right now, she's in the playground. Has she had a snack? Has she got any friends to play with? Is she OK? Is she happy? This dislocated sense of being bodily present at work, yet with your heart beating elsewhere is a feeling many of us will recognize.

I remember reading an article by Anne-Marie Slaughter, director of policy planning in the State Department under the Obama administration and the first woman to hold that post. It was titled 'Why Women Still Can't Have It All'.[23] In it, she describes her own tipping point, when she no longer felt she could have it all. 'President and Mrs Obama hosted a glamorous reception . . . I sipped champagne, greeted foreign dignitaries, and mingled. But I could not stop thinking about my 14-year-old son, who [was] skipping homework, disrupting classes, failing math, and tuning out any adult who tried to reach him.'

Slaughter felt it, too, the heart tug. The emotional pivot from work to home. It was a big deal, to me, reading this. An impressive woman saying: this job – a job most of us could only dream of – simply doesn't work for me at this particular moment. Sometimes you can go for it. Sometimes you just can't.

She exposed the cracks when she admitted, 'How unexpectedly hard it was to do the kind of job I wanted to do as a high government official and be the kind of parent I wanted to be, at a demanding time for my children.' Slaughter left the job because it didn't allow her to go *with* the grain of life. It required her to put the blinkers on and power through, regardless of what was happening behind the scenes.

This brings me to flex. Home life has its own rhythm, its ebbs and flows. When we embrace flex, we acknowledge those fluctuations. For me, it was my daughter starting school. For Slaughter, it was her teenager going through a tough time. But it could be anything. An elderly parent who has had a fall or a partner's new commute that creates havoc for school drop-offs. It may be that you are moving home, having health problems or going through a relationship break-up. The tug of home life can be intense at these times; at others it can be imperceptible. Shutting the front door when you leave for work can sometimes feel like an escape. But sometimes, it feels like abandonment.

It's so easy to see success in terms of career, a job title, a salary rise. But the home is a neglected part of this conversation. Home needs our attention; it needs to feel joyful, it needs to feel happy and balanced. As I will show in this chapter, very often all of this falls on women's shoulders. And it shouldn't. Our partners also need to think about career ambitions, working hours, chores in the home, childcare and how all of this might flex around the needs of the people in their life.

Home life has its own
rhythm, its ebbs and
flows. When we embrace
flex, we acknowledge
those fluctuations.

Here, I will look at how gender relationships in the home are flexing. And I will explain how to spread and share responsibilities in the home and outside of it. This chapter will give you the checklists to be more intentional about your roles. It aims to help you ensure you're not pulled in too many different directions or left carrying the emotional load, which is the invisible – and unrewarded – work of managing the needs of the entire household. And it will give you the conversation starters to have the difficult chats.

WOMEN'S EMOTIONAL LOAD: COPING WITH THE TICKER TAPE

In the past, roles were clearer. The template was man as breadwinner and woman as homemaker. This still absolutely exists and works for many couples, but it is no longer the norm.

Today, the household comes in all different shapes and sizes. No kids, single parent, two dads or two mums, mum as breadwinner and stay-at-home dad, blended families, dual income families, beanpole families with more than two generations under one roof – take your pick. The modern family is diverse, impossible to pigeonhole, messy and beautiful.

And roles within the home are blurring. Over the last half century, in the majority of countries and across all income levels, the number of women working is higher than three decades ago.[24]

Most studies report that men are spending more time with their children. Nearly three-quarters of the British public now disagrees with the attitude that women should look after the home while men earn a living. But who does what in the home? That seems to be less clear cut. With more of us working, with more on everyone's plate, who is keeping the home running?

There are loads of brilliant men out there, doing their share. But the short answer is women. Despite all these societal shifts, so much of work and management of the home still lies with us. Take one of the most mundane and seemingly innocuous parts of life. It's a bellwether for gender equality and a tinder-box to marital relations.

Housework.

The 'housework gap' between men and women stopped narrowing back in the late 1990s (until then, women were gradually decreasing the time they spent doing housework as men increased theirs). When it comes to unpaid chores at home, the Office for National Statistics found in 2016 that women do almost 40 per cent more than men. [25]

Types of chores are split along gender lines. Women tend to do daily tasks like childcare, laundry, cooking and cleaning. Men tend to do outdoor chores such as car maintenance and gardening. So, the stuff that needs doing about once a week or less.

So far, so unsurprising. But when we dig into the research, the picture gets a little more complicated.

For a start, same-sex couples are better at chore equality than straight couples. More same-sex, dual-earner couples share laundry and household repair than straight couples. And same-sex couples were much more likely to share childcare equally (74 per cent of gay couples versus 38 per cent of straight couples). A lesson could be learned from this – neither one is doing the traditional role of

THE IKUMEN PROJECT

In Japan, with its history of salarymen and long working hours, a fascinating cultural change is taking place. The Japanese government, faced with falling birthrates and an ageing population, tried to understand why being a mum was less appealing to women. They assumed women felt conflicted about their careers. But they were wrong. Women were avoiding motherhood because they knew their male partners wouldn't do anything to help. But men weren't shirking child-rearing out of sexism or laziness. When surveyed in 2008, a third of working fathers wanted to spend more time with their children and to take paternity leave, but felt their bosses would disapprove.

So the government started the 'Ikumen Project' (a melding of Japanese *ikuji*, meaning 'child-rearing', and the English 'men') with the objective of getting more men involved in bringing up children and making workplaces dad-friendly. In 2009, advertising agency Dentsu invented the term *papa danshi* – 'papa men' – to try and make fathers who are 'highly motivated in child-rearing' cool. It seemed to work. By 2015, the percentage of men who took paternity leave increased from 1.9 per cent in 2012 to nearly 3 per cent in 2015 and 7 per cent in 2017. These are not groundbreaking figures, but the seeds of cultural change seem to be planted. [26]

'mum/wife' or 'dad/husband'. They are both mucking in and figuring it out, free from gendered expectations of how things 'should' be divided.

I love the example of 'mommunes', as they are known in America: a group of single mothers and their children sharing one home, supporting each other, creating a new kind of family unit and dividing up chores between them. One example in the UK is Janet, Vicky and Nicola's set-up in south London. As one of the three mums describe it: 'It was like a marriage, only better. We had a kind of invisible rota. We cooked proper dinners for each other every night. We had roles.' Janet did the paperwork. Vicky baked. Nicola cooked Sunday dinners and, she says, cleaned up after parties.[27] This is another example of a non-traditional approach that came from experimenting and adapting to each other's strengths.

None of this is easy, mind. A lawyer friend told me about her set-up: she is the bread-winner and her partner is at home with the four kids. She stresses the time it took to adapt to these roles. 'It was two years of hell adjusting to working while he looked after the kids and house ALL WRONG. We had to gradually let go of gender roles.' The people around them needed to let go of them too. 'The mums at the school insist on setting up after-school stuff with me. "Er, I'm in court. I don't know whether the kid can play on Tuesday. Ask his dad."' And others questioned whether their relationship would be affected. 'People always used to say, "Oh, don't you/he find the fact he doesn't have a job emasculating?" To which my standard response was, "No, he's got a massive dick." True or untrue, it did the job of shutting them up.'

It's clearly not as simple as swapping roles.

Women who out-earn their partners still do more work in the home. Nearly three-quarters of Americans expect women to have the primary responsibility for cooking at home – even if they spend the same amount of time at work and make more money than their husbands.[28]

And the more they out-earn their partners, the less he is willing to do! There is evidence to suggest in households where the woman is the breadwinner, the more she earns, the less he does in the house. It is as though she is being punished for out-earning her partner. As the author of one study put it: 'We can imagine these men thinking, "She might earn all the money, but I'm not going to do dishes."'[29]

I double-take when I read this. Dishes are really interesting when it comes to gender roles in the home.

In the research I've read, what's the task which breaks the camel's back? Washing dishes. Women who say they wash the majority of dishes report 'significantly more relationship discord, lower relationship satisfaction, and less sexual satisfaction than women who split the dishes with their partner'.[30] Hold up – less sexual satisfaction? Men, get the Fairy liquid out. Washing dishes can improve your sex life, it's official.

It's not just sexual satisfaction that is compromised; it's women's time too. Women get over 4.5 fewer hours of leisure time per week than men.[31] That free time is eaten up by housework as we've seen – but not only that. A huge amount of list-making, planning and choreographing goes on under the surface, essential to keeping a busy home life flowing.

Washing dishes can
improve your sex life,
it's official.

This week for example, I have a ticker tape of tasks hovering on the periphery of my vision:

>> Birthday present for my nephew >> New baby card for my cousin >> Cling film >> Dentist appointments for all of us >> Haircut for daughter no. 1 >> Call friend in Hong Kong >> Check how mum's mole removal went >> Fix dripping tap >> Give the dog more love >> Sellotape>>

This is known as the emotional load: the unrecognized and unrewarded work that keeps a household running. Managing the emotional load requires great skill. Foresight – knowing that there's a birthday party at the weekend, and the present cupboard is bare. Detail – noticing the children's toenails have become talons and they need de-clawing. Delegation – can Grandma do the school pick-up if we're both working late? Empathy – a friend is going through a divorce, pick up the phone, drop round, be there.

Most of the time, the emotional load is on women's shoulders. One mum told me she doubted her husband even knew which school year her kids were in. Just as we are conditioned to see housework as something suited to women's character, the emotional load is seen as intrinsically female.

It's not. It's just that women are brought up to believe we are better at all of this. Women, we're told, are born nurturers, with natural intuition and empathy.

Society tells us a good woman has her emotional antennae continually quivering, alert to every need of the people surrounding her. In the home, she anticipates, she plans, she remembers, she multitasks – and all of this gives men a pass to be emotionally lazy. None of this is innately female, but it's work that women have absorbed into their lives – so much so that men might be unaware of it going on around them.

The emotional load isn't just made up of booking plumbers and buying birthday cards. During sex, women are still on duty – seemingly giving more attention to their partner's ego than their own pleasure. A study found that 79 per cent of women faked an orgasm half of the times they had sex, with the majority believing it boosted their partner's self-esteem (which is why they were doing it in the first place). [32]

Add >> fake orgasm >> boost his mojo >> to that never-ending ticker tape . . .

Our leisure time is depleted and, with this constant management of all the emotions that surround us, so is our mental bandwidth. Imagine the ideas and creativity that could burst free if only we weren't thinking about the dog's worming tablets. Imagine the energy we could give to our families, our friends, our careers and our health. Imagine our sex lives, if only someone else washed the bloody dishes.

We need to look closely at the home and flex these gendered roles, lighten the emotional load, free up our bandwidth and re-channel our energy. Otherwise we're curbing our own potential.

HOW TO FLEX RELATIONSHIPS & ROLES IN THE HOME

One of the UK's power couples, Justine Roberts, CEO of Mumsnet, and her husband Ian Katz, director of programmes at Channel 4, examined a list of all their responsibilities in the home on a spreadsheet. Both have big jobs and both are equally pressurized outside the home. But when counting their tasks inside the home, Justine had 65 and Ian had 5 (one of his was lightbulbs, and she commented how often they ended up sitting in the dark). She said: 'We had a conversation about how we could go about getting a more equal division of labour and he agrees in principle, but it's the practice you have to keep on at.'[33]

For a practical solution, look to the Everyday Sexism Project Chore Challenge. They asked couples to keep a two-week log of all the chores (the physical and the emotional) that they do in the home and then gender swap them.

This might seem extreme. But you could start with just writing down the ticker tape for this week and discussing how to share the work. The process of documenting all the work that needs to get done, logging the emotional load and having the conversation to allocate those jobs is the first start to flexing your roles.

The next priority is to work out who does what. If one person is doing everything and the other person is doing nothing, the relationship will suffer. But tasks don't have to be strictly equal to impact couple satisfaction. It's more important that each individual is clear about their responsibilities, content with their share and feels like they are making an active choice. Satisfaction is driven more by whether couples talk about how to divide responsibilities than in the precise division of household tasks. We are much more likely to be unsatisfied, or even resentful, if we stay silent instead of voicing our wishes earlier in the relationship.

Clichés of women being better at talking about their issues than men should be banished. A study of 225 couples in the US found that gay men in partnerships were much more likely to say they had discussed how to divide the household labour when they first moved in together. Women in straight partnerships were much more likely to say they wanted to, but didn't (and were therefore more unhappy with their domestic arrangements).[34]

So, you've written it down, you've discussed who does what, but don't fall into the trap of having to beg for help every time something needs doing.

The emotional load isn't really lifted if you are compiling lists, micro-managing the tasks and then asking politely for someone else to do them. It's still on you – you're still the one conducting the boring chore orchestra (the chore-chestra? The bore-chestra?). Perhaps we'll never have true equality until we're all equally bored.

And regarding equality, try and model it for your children. Children scrutinize their parents all the time. They have Sherlock Holmes-like powers of observation. If you have children, be conscious that you are creating templates for them. What are we revealing about our faith in men when we mock 'Daddy day care'? What does it say to kids when fathers say they are 'babysitting' their own children when Mum goes out? If we want to change gender stereotypes for the next generation, it needs to start with us.

If we want to change gender stereotypes for the next generation, it needs to start with us.

Be aware that men tend to do the outdoor chores that are infrequent and women tend to do everything else. Try and mix it up. Dad, pack for the holidays. Mum, take out the bins. Everything might fall apart, but who knows, it might not and your kids will dislodge their assumptions and expect the load to be shared when they grow up.

CREATE A
JOINT VISION

Of course, flexing the home isn't just about the chores. It's about creating a joint vision of the lives we want to live, our career goals, and how that will work over time. We need to think carefully about when we accelerate at work and when we consolidate and slow down. When we do this, we take control.

Avivah Wittenberg-Cox, gender expert and author of *How Women Mean Business*, advocates big-picture thinking. She thinks that it should be less about the jigsaw puzzle of two different careers and more about designing a life together. She asks: 'What's the life that we want to build? What are our goals, our mission?

What are we going to prioritize, when? Is it family, is it money, is it impact?' Within that framework, where do we flex around each other's ambitions and needs?

One way of thinking about this is the '*Borgen* model'. *Borgen* is a Danish political drama television series which aired in the UK in 2012. My friends and I became obsessed with it, in particular the Birgitte Nyborg character, who became the first female prime minister of Denmark. In the series, she had an agreement with her husband Philip, an academic, that she would have the 'lead career' for five years as prime minister, whilst his career took a back seat and he managed the emotional load, looking after the kids and the home. After this, she would step back and give him his turn. Despite it not quite going to plan, I loved this arrangement and found it inspiring. The generosity of making trade-offs for one other, and seeing a bigger picture of joint and intertwined success seemed like a revelation. It is also a bold and proactive approach, rather than just fire-fighting in response to opportunities or problems.

Now, this need not be a five-year set-in-stone contract. It could be a looser agreement to flex around each other's ambitions.

SHARERS VS WINNERS

Not everyone is willing to give the *Borgen* model a go.
A study of 42 heterosexual men in mostly dual earner couples
who worked at a global strategy consulting firm exposed
stark differences in the men's willingness to flex around their
partner's careers. The study divided them into two groups:
– the 'breadsharers': men who believed their wives should
  equally pursue their work and family goals.
  the 'breadwinners': men who attached low social status
  to their wives' professions.

The breadsharers were more likely to be open to flexing their
own careers and changing jobs, cities or countries if that might
be needed in the future for their wife's career. A typical quote
was: 'I want to make sure she continues to be in a professional
situation where she can [succeed], and that . . . puts pressure
back on me to . . . say, "OK, wait. Our life is not going to be the
one where I get to do whatever I want job-wise, just because my
life is not the centre."'

The breadwinners intended to stay at the firm and try their
hardest to make partner, and were not willing to flex around
their wives' careers. A breadwinner quote: 'She could have done
much more than she has [in her field], but she chose a different
path. What I call, you know — being a project manager in the
home . . .' Bear in mind, in this instance, his wife's salary made
up one third of the family's income! You can only flex your home
if you have a partner who is open to it. [35]

HELEN DWYER'S FLEX STORY

*Helen Dwyer, 63, is a retired school principal
in Bathurst, Australia*

I left school at the age of 17. I took up any retail work
I could get, met my husband-to-be and generally had
a good time and 'fun in the sun' life. I was married at 20 and
by the time I was 32 had two children (two and six years old),
was virtually working full-time in between a news agency,
bakery and handbag store whilst my husband worked full-time
shift work.

At this stage, my husband and I had a conversation and
both decided that I should apply for university to study for a
teaching diploma. We felt this would be a good move to allow
us a better lifestyle and a more secure future for our family.

It meant we juggled the care of our children, had a
mortgage and lived from week to week. Over the three years it
took to gain my qualifications, my husband continued to work
shift work and I continued to work part-time. Between us we
cared for our children.

We had no family support where we lived, so it really was up
to us to work as a team. The childcare was a constant juggle.
My eldest, Luke, had started school and my youngest Gareth
was two when I started university. I was able to secure one day
per week at the university daycare for Gareth which was not

flexible. I would keep my fingers crossed each semester and try to get as much uni or library time in on that day. I had a great neighbour who would care for Gareth and Luke after school in the gaps. Work was important for both of us due to the cost of the care for Gareth, uni costs
and the cost of living.

None of this ever went smoothly! Often we were problem-solving on the run – things like illness (kids, carers or us), timetabling changes at uni, extra shifts at work and unexpected things that pop up in life. Also, I had six practical assessments in schools over the three years, which would throw everything out. My mother-in-law – God bless her – would leave her home to stay with us for these times.

It paid off as I graduated from university with distinction, as one of the top 10 graduates in my year, and was rewarded with a full-time teaching position with the New South Wales Department of Education.

Fortunately, all of this was a shared goal with my husband. If it wasn't, I would never have achieved it. We were able to live a more comfortable and secure life with our children, and my husband was then able to pursue goals of his own. Our children were able to follow their interests with our support. I recently retired as a school principal after a wonderful and fulfilling career in education spanning 27 years.

And that brings us on to the final point. A friend who leads a big institution in the public sector says his staff (often women) are increasingly coming to him with requests for more flexible working. He is pleased that these conversations are happening, but he questions whether, in some instances, flexible working will solve the deeper problems at play.

'People come to me and talk about flex, and I want to say go and talk to your husband. The conversation should start at home.' In some of these instances, the woman is bending her career and her life around an intractable male partner's job, or his refusal to take on any of the domestic load. She is flexing, but is progress really being made?

We should flex, but we shouldn't become contortionists, bending over backwards. And we all need to start the conversation at home.

We should flex,
but we shouldn't become
contortionists, bending
over backwards.
And we all need to start
the conversation at
home.

HOW TO FLEX
YOUR HOME

~

1. Write down all the chores that are done in the home.
    In Excel if you're fancy, on the back of an unopened
    bill if you're not. Be awe-inspired at the amount you
    are currently doing. Be shocked at how little anyone
    else is doing.

2. Allocate some time with your partner to discuss
    who does what. You could start by working through
    each room of the house and noting jobs associated
    with that room. You could then think in terms of
    tasks that are daily (cooking, cleaning, childcare);
    weekly (food shop, scheduling playdates), and yearly
    (purchasing insurance, the car's MOT). It's not about
    a 50/50 divide. It's about being happy with your lot.

3. Be sensitive. This conversation may be fraught,
    especially if either party feels resentful at the amount
    they are currently doing. A good way to approach
    things would be to appreciate and acknowledge
    what each of you is doing before explaining what you
    would like help with. Then negotiate. You may hate

doing the laundry but not mind doing the hoovering. Could you use that as a bargaining tool?

4. Model good behaviours for your children so they don't just associate women with home and men with work. Men: mop floors. Women: mow the lawn.

5. Don't micro-manage the to-do list, or feel like you need to beg for help each time something needs doing. Don't end up being the 'conductor of the chore chestra'. Encourage your partner to proactively take responsibility for a whole task area. For example, whoever is in charge of school shoes needs to know the children's shoe size, when they've grown out of them and arrange to buy new ones.

6. Discuss a longer-term vision of the lives you want to live and work out priorities within that. How can you and your partner flex around each other? Think about the *Borgen* model. Might it work for you? What other model could work?

SUMMARY

Flex is more than a band-aid solution to see you through changing times at home. Permission to flex between home and work is liberating. Permission to define success in the way we want to – whether it is raising a family or raising hell at work – is liberating.

We need to turn our attention to what is happening inside our homes, relationships and families. The modern household looks and feels different from the one we grew up in. Roles within it are less defined, and day-to-day life feels more complex. We add more and more items to our mental ticker tapes. We're negotiating gender roles, both in the home and outside, which means that everything is up for grabs.

We need to be OK with that and take inspiration from pioneering non-traditional units, like mommunes, gay couples and stay-at-home dads. By creating new models and forging new paths, they are paving the way for the households of the future. Like them, we need to experiment, to invent, to work out what kind of life we really want to live with the people who are most precious to us. We should think about how best to achieve that, together. We need to talk it through, because things are changing under our noses. Work is important, but home matters the most, and just because our roles and relationships are bending, they don't need to break.

'We need to reshape
our own perception of
how we view ourselves.
We have to step up as
women and take
the lead.'

BEYONCÉ

FLEX

~

& THE

~

BODY

When I talk about flex and the body, I'm not referring to exercise and stretching (although I highly approve of both). This chapter is less about the ability to touch your toes, and more about the skill of really listening to your body and flexing your life to work *with* it, rather than *against* it.

It's only recently I started listening to my body. For most of my adult life, I treated it as a sort of machine to propel me through life. Sometimes the machine fired on all cylinders, but at other times it ground to a halt and I grew impatient. I drank an extra coffee if I felt tired, I dosed up with Lemsip if a cold was brewing, I took a painkiller when I had menstrual cramps.

Forcing myself to carry on as normal, whilst practical and sometimes necessary in the short term, doesn't work for me any more. It ignores my body's rhythms, moods and cycles. It meant I ended up doing things like writing a detailed report when my brain was distracted (resulting in tea breaks, Twitter binges, muddled thinking and little work). Or throwing a party when I'm at my most insecure (take it from me – hermit-like host plus awkward guests is not a recipe for fun times). So I started to realize that ignoring my body is not very smart.

"

Sometimes, it ain't
exactly broke, but it does
need fixing.

"

Much of my body-as-machine attitude is inherited. My parents have a rigid approach to health. You are either at death's door, or you need to pull your socks up and get on with it. For them, doctors are quacks and catastrophe-mongers, and should be avoided at all costs. On health, their mantra is 'if it ain't broke, don't fix it'.

But sometimes, it ain't exactly broke, but it does need fixing. When I was 37, I felt exhausted most of the time. I had two little girls under the age of six. I didn't really exercise, unless you counted the speed walking I did around London every day to get to the train station, to the office, to the nursery. I slept terribly, falling into an exhausted slump by 10 p.m. every night only to awake at 3 a.m. with creeping dread. My washing-machine brain churned over fragments of my day, which were perfectly ordinary but in the lonely pre-dawn seemed filled with menace. I realized something had to change, and for me that was sleep.

Sleep is such a mysterious part of life. Every one of us, on average, will sleep 24 years in our lifetime. That's 24 years of dreams we forget. Twenty-four years of repair and restoration which we take for granted. Twenty-four years of inhaled flies and drool-soaked pillows. If we have a lifelong partner, that's likely to be a good ten years of shared slumber, unconscious battles over duvets, tender, intertwined limbs, and fogs of morning breath. We take no notice of this huge chunk of our lives, until it evades us.

My insomnia was a message from my body I couldn't ignore. I made a decision then, aged 37, that I was going to address my sleep issues. It started me on a different journey, that of understanding my body more holistically.

In this chapter, I examine two areas of women's lives which often get neglected – sleep and periods. The better we understand them, and our rhythms and moods, the better we are able to flex our schedules and our expectations so that we can perform at our best and happiest.

THIS IS THE RHYTHM OF THE NIGHT: UNDERSTANDING YOUR BODY CLOCK

Our body clocks are governed by circadian rhythms – physical, mental and behavioural patterns that follow a 24-hour cycle: *circum* means 'around', *dies* means 'day'. The average rhythm during a day is that we warm up and reach peak alertness at around noon. This peak then decreases until about 3 p.m. – the slump when we usually reach for a cup of tea, a snack or a can of cola. In some parts of the world, like Spain, this is the time when people take a siesta. After this trough, our alertness tends to climb towards a second high at around 6 p.m. Then it's a steady decline to 3.30 a.m. After this, alertness climbs again and the cycle repeats the following day.

Bizarre then, that peak alertness for the average person comes at noon, just when we're about to head off to lunch, and at 6 p.m., when we're probably commuting home. In terms of the standard work day at least, this can represent a huge lost opportunity.

However, individuals do vary in their patterns of alertness. Some of us have a genetic predisposition to function really well in the morning ('larks') or perform better in the evening ('owls'). Those who fall somewhere in between, and relate to the average rhythm, are 'hummingbirds'. This is your chronotype: your body's natural timeline for eating, sleeping and working.

I'm probably the lovechild of a hummingbird and an owl (a howl?). If my children didn't wake me up every day at 6:30 a.m. I'd happily sleep until 9 a.m. As it stands, I'm groggy and slow in the mornings. On the Tube in the morning rush hour, jammed into someone's armpit, I take refuge in headphones and coffee. Between the hours of 10 a.m. and noon I'm on fire. This is when I feel efficient, creative and shit gets done. Shit stops at 12:30 p.m. when I'm suddenly ravenous. After lunch, I chug along nicely until about four when I slip into first gear. If I'm at work, I need a cup of a tea and a chat about my latest podcast obsession. If I'm at home I need to stand in front of the fridge eating handfuls of cheese. Post-cheese, there's another mini peak (a fun conversation over dinner, or I might dive into some efficient work) before bed at 11 p.m.

Whether you are a lark, an owl or a hummingbird is driven by differing levels of the two hormones involved in regulating sleep. Cortisol rises in the morning and powers us to wake up. Melatonin increases in the evening and helps wind our bodies down for sleep. For night owls, melatonin rises later in the day than the average, while cortisol increases earlier than average for morning larks.

And this doesn't remain stable – our body clocks change throughout our lives. As a child enters teenage years, pubertal hormones shift the body clock by one to two hours, which means teens become owl-ish, and naturally sleep and wake later during adolescence. Blamed for being lazy, teens are actually just adapting to a new rhythm of their body clock. Teens need about eight to ten hours of sleep each night to function best. And because they are falling asleep later, but still having to get up at the same time for school, most teens are sleep-deprived – one study found that only 15 per cent reported sleeping eight and a half hours on school nights.[36]

How many of us remember those teenage mornings of feeling exhausted and grumpy? How many of us are now coping with teens who need to be prised out of bed? Life today, with its dominant rhythm of 9–5 p.m. for workers and 8.30 a.m. to 4 p.m. for students, is better suited to larks. Owls build up a sleep debt over time which results in health issues; owls have higher rates of depression and anxiety.

For night-shift workers, this is amplified. As well the health fallout from irregular eating habits and interrupted sleep, they can also feel out of sync with their loved ones, which may chip away at their wellbeing.

An owl friend who is also a shift worker talks of her dislocation from her friends. When she meets them for a meal, she isn't hungry at the right time. When she wants to chat, they are going to bed. I often wake up to a bunch of WhatsApp messages she sends me overnight – we are in different emotional time zones, desperate to get onto the same page.

We should do as much as possible to flex our activities to fit with the natural circadian rhythms of the day, and our chronotype within that. The timetables of those doing night-shift work will be very different, and flexing work hours may not be possible in all industries. But what follows are some thoughts on how you might be able to flex your days and weeks to work with your natural body clock.

ARE YOU A LARK, OWL OR A HUMMINGBIRD?

~ Decide your chronotype – in other words, whether you are a lark or an owl or a bit of both. Around 10 per cent of us are larks and 20 per cent are owls – the rest of us, known as hummingbirds, fall somewhere in between.
~ Larks tend to sleep between the hours of 10 p.m. and 6 a.m., or earlier. Larks find it hard to sleep in, even if they have gone to bed later. Peak productivity is around noon and they fizzle out in the early evening.
~ Owls tend to stay awake until past midnight, and would wake after 10 a.m. if they could. Peak productivity is the middle of the day and the evening.
~ Hummingbirds wake up at 7 a.m. and go to bed around 11 p.m. They tend to be alert throughout the average nine-to-five day but slump in the early afternoon.

TIPS FOR LARKS

~ Larks can fit in morning exercise before the day
  gets started.
~ Larks are great at doing the school run calmly, getting
  everyone out the door and on time to school, whereas
  other chronotypes might find it pressurized and fraught.
~ Larks should do their most challenging work first
  thing. Avoid distractions in the late morning around
  your noon peak. Can you switch off emails until the
  afternoon, which will allow you to focus, undistracted?
~ Think about a mid-morning snack to keep you going
  at 10 a.m.
~ Larks should do their more routine work – answering
  emails and non-demanding admin, for example – in
  the afternoon.
~ Arrange social activities over lunch and coffees in the
  week, so you're not pushing yourself to be fun when
  you'd rather be curled up in bed with a book.
~ Larks should begin winding down at 9.30 p.m.
  and turn off all screens. The blue light from devices
  activates your brain and makes it harder to go to sleep.
~ If possible, can you flex your working day to start at
  7 a.m. and finish at 3 p.m.?

TIPS FOR OWLS

~ Owls will be rushed in the morning. Can you pack school bags or set out clothes for the next day the night before?

~ Could you also make your breakfast the previous evening? That way you won't miss breakfast or have to flap about when you are half asleep.

~ If at work, use the morning for routine work and planning – answer emails, write lists, plan ahead.

~ Try not to schedule meetings or socialize before lunch, when you might still be in first gear.

~ Owls should do their difficult, most brain-taxing work after lunch.

~ Owls should think about flexing around the second peak at about 6 p.m. If you can leave later and miss commuter rush hour, you could achieve great things in a focused period in the early evening. The benefit is that everyone else will have gone home, so the email flow should slow down, giving you undistracted time.

~ Find a time to work out after 6 p.m., when you're most energetic.

~ If possible, can you flex your working day to start at 11 a.m. and finish at 7 p.m.?

TIPS FOR HUMMINGBIRDS

~ The nine-to-five is best suited to the hummingbird.
~ Peak productivity is at noon – a good time for 30
  minutes of concentrated work, a workout or blitzing
  some housework.
~ Have a snack at about 3 p.m., when you might need
  a pick-me-up.
~ If you have problems sleeping, avoid foods rich in fat
  or sugar late at night as these will be difficult to digest.
~ If you tend to potter around in the late evening and
  find it hard to wind down, consider setting an alarm
  to remind you to go to bed.

Sleep is the magic formula for a better life. The first
thing we need to do is value it and make sure we get
enough of it. Scientists have shown that a good night's
sleep leads to happier, more creative, longer lives. But we
can go further than that. Tweaking your daily activities
to fit your chronotype means you can personalize your
routine and live and work at your best. When I began
to understand my sleep rhythms it was a revelation.
The next rhythm I wanted to understand was my
menstrual cycle.

ABOUT BLOODY TIME: UNDERSTANDING PERIODS

My generation was taught to associate periods with shame. We were not to talk about them, to hide tampons up our sleeves on our way to the toilet and to see bleeding as messy and inconvenient. It was a female zone, not fit for male attention or conversation.

Even the language we used showed shame. Go to a chemist and you'd see shelves of 'feminine hygiene' or 'sanitary products' – arguably male language to describe a natural process which is neither unhygienic nor unsanitary.

Menstrual advertising coyly showed blue liquid, as though blood was too disgusting to acknowledge. The message from these ads was loud and clear. They said: 'We get you. We get those damn inconvenient, unpleasant, embarrassing periods. Don't worry, we've got your back (and by "your back", we mean your gusset). We'll get you back to normal again (and by "normal", we mean rollerblading and kitesurfing).'

But I didn't want to get back to normal. I WAS normal. It *is* normal to bleed every month, so why were we in a state of frenzied, shameful denial?

Before we can flex around our periods, the first thing we have to do is talk about them. And this is starting to happen. A de-shaming revolution is happening, and periods have risen on the cultural agenda. Period poverty is a campaigning hotspot, with people like 18-year-old north London schoolgirl and founder of #FreePeriods Amika George campaigning for girls who qualify for free school meals to also get free menstrual products.

More recent menstrual product advertising has started to tackle some bold topics. Bodyform was the first brand to show blood in adverts instead of the industry standard of blue liquid in their 'Blood Normal' campaign.

Businesses and governments have begun to respond too. Nike has had menstrual leave in their code of conduct since 2007. In some countries, governmental legislation offering menstrual leave exists already, yet take-up is low as women fear they will be judged and their chances of promotion will fall. But what is the point of legislation if women don't benefit from it? Periods are still a source of shame.

Talking about them at work is still seen as detrimental to your professionalism. Who amongst us would approach a possibly male boss, tampon in hand and say: 'I'm cramping with period pain, I'm bleeding like a bastard so I'm off home to down some Nurofen and watch Netflix in bed.'

Dr Jan Toledano, a specialist at the London Hormone Clinic, agrees. 'Society is not very forgiving and women are expected to fit in with the workplace. There is massive pressure for women to carry on as usual despite their symptoms.'

MENSTRUAL LEAVE AROUND THE WORLD

Menstrual leave has been a legal right for Japanese women since 1947, granting women with period pain *seirikyuuka* or 'psychological leave'. South Korea introduced a law in 2001 that allows women to take one day of menstrual leave per month. In 2016, the Chinese province of Anhui became the third Chinese province to introduce period leave, allowing women with severe menstrual pain to take one to two days every month, on presenting a doctor's certificate.

The fact remains that before we can begin to flex around our cycles, we need to change the conversation around periods and break the taboos.

All around us, the conversation about periods is changing. It's a crucial topic for Flex. Throughout our cycles, hormone levels fluctuate making us feel, behave and perform differently as we move through the month. The changes in levels of progesterone and oestrogen affect brain cognition, emotions, sensory processing and appetite (as well as the performance-related aspects Emma Hayes mentions on page 132). It makes sense to lean into these changes, rather than fear them. If we adjust our routines, social lives and work behaviours to suit our bodies, it stands to reason we could feel, live and work better.

This is called cycle syncing. Understanding your cycle and adjusting life to suit it is a form of self-care, of being kind to yourself. Can you put yourself forward for the activities and social engagements that will make you feel happy and fulfilled rather than inhibited and like you're failing?

TABOO-BREAKING IN SPORT

The conversation around periods is changing in the traditionally macho world of sport. Serena Williams was at the frontier back in 2005 when she talked about her menstrual migraines. In 2015, British tennis player Heather Watson talked – euphemistically, but at least she spoke up – of 'girl things' when she was beaten in the Australian Open, and Kiran Gandhi, drummer for British-Sri Lankan rapper M.I.A., ran the London Marathon whilst on her period 'free-bleeding', using no menstrual product, with blood running down her legs.

In women's football in the UK, Emma Hayes was the coach of Chelsea Ladies when they won the League and FA Cup double in 2018. She has studied the impact of menstrual cycles on players' reaction times, manual dexterity, neuromuscular co-ordination, blood sugar levels and muscle maintenance.

'This subject is pushed away like a taboo but it's important,' Hayes says. 'If I had unlimited resources, I would hire someone to manage my players' menstrual cycles.'[37] Imagine the 'marginal gains' that could be made by analysing the team's cycles and changing game plans accordingly. If male athletes had periods, there would be teams of people researching and monitoring them. Understanding the physiological and emotional impact of cycles could be a game-changer outside of sport, too. If we can flex our personal game plans to sync with our cycles, it could help us achieve our own peak performance.

GO WITH
YOUR FLOW

'Everyone has a different cycle,' says Toledano. 'Some don't have any symptoms at all but some are quite incapacitated, which can last half the month. This can impact cognitive function which affects work. We can feel clumsy, foggy – we can't think straight.'

I relate to this. My mental and emotional state changes throughout my cycle. At some points, I feel confident, extrovert and my mood is buoyant. But nearing my period, I can feel anxious, inhibited and tend to catastrophize. An unanswered WhatsApp translates to 'my friend hates me'. My daughter's tummy ache sends me scrambling to Dr Google for terrifying possible diagnoses. It took until my late thirties to spot the patterns in these feelings, and see them as cyclical rather than permanent personality traits. I used a period tracking app to document my symptoms and feelings, and gradually I became able to anticipate moods and actually flex my life around my cycle. And I'm not alone. The rise of period tracking apps like Clue and Flow are testament to an appetite to understand our bodies and cycles better.

If you are someone who menstruates, try tracking your symptoms using an app, or just on paper, to note how you are feeling both physically and emotionally, and start to adjust your plans. Remember that every body is different; some people who menstruate have a 35-day cycle, others a 24-day cycle, and things are different again if you are on the Pill or are experiencing the menopause.

HOW TO FLEX
WITH YOUR CYCLE

One way to understand your menstrual cycle is to think of the four phases as seasons, as Kate Shepherd Cohen does, and try to flex your activities around those seasons.

1. **Winter: Menstrual phase (days 1 to 7)**

BODY: Your oestrogen and progesterone levels are low, your uterus sheds its lining. You are on your period. At this time, you bleed and you might experience backache, tiredness and food cravings. Testosterone production boosts sex drive during the period.

MIND: You might feel knackered, withdrawn and antisocial. Rather than forcing yourself to plod on as usual, this is your cue to look after yourself and conserve energy. See this time as a treat and a retreat from the crazed pace of everyday life. An overloaded schedule is likely to push you over the edge. Learn to say no, elegantly. Enjoy going for walks, reading and making delicious meals. You might watch box sets or have lots of sex, riding the wave of high libido. Might be hard to do both, depending on how good the box set is.

2. Spring: Follicular phase (days 8 to 13)

BODY: In this phase, your body is preparing to ovulate (release an egg). Your oestrogen levels start to increase from their decline in the menstrual phase, and your uterus lining builds up with blood, tissue and nutrients to prepare for implantation of the fertilized egg.

MIND: As oestrogen levels rise, you may be buzzing, physically energized, mentally alert and positive about the future. It's a fresh start. At work, you're on fire. You are smart and productive. You say clever things and resist the urge to mic drop when you leave a room. You learn quicker, so it's a great time for creativity and gaining new skills. See this time as a procrastination killer, start something you've been putting off. 'Spring' is for risk-taking and pushing your boundaries – you're in the zone.

3. **Summer: Ovulatory phase (Days 14 to 21)**

BODY: Ovulation begins. The egg is released on its journey down the fallopian tube. If it meets sperm on this journey, it will become fertilized. Oestrogen levels are peaking and testosterone also rises. You may feel pelvic pain or twinges – this has a lovely name for something so unlovely: Mittelschmerz, the German for 'middle pain'. You may experience bloating and painful boobs.

MIND: High oestrogen makes you bolder, more confident and ready for a challenge. Social skills are at their highest – you are super-fun. New friends think you're the bee's knees, old friends remember why they liked you in the first place. Testosterone also rises, which means you can feel more impulsive, daring and competitive. And when testosterone spikes, it boosts your libido. See this as a phase for socializing, sex and super-powers.

4. **Autumn: Luteal phase (Days 22 to 28)**

BODY: Oestrogen levels drop off during this phase and progesterone increases. You could experience PMS symptoms like acne, sleep disturbances, mood changes and cramping.

MIND: Progesterone is a sedating, anti-anxiety hormone. You might feel brooding and cautious. You might have bouts of sadness or crying. You might want to be surrounded by close friends who love and understand you, or you may want to hide from the world. Your brain is primed for detail rather than big-picture thinking. See 'Autumn' as a time to slow down, get your life in order and plan. Winter is coming, friends. Winter is coming.

SUMMARY

We should delight in the body rather than fear it; listen to it rather than ignore it. We should talk about our cycles and mood fluctuations rather than feeling ashamed of them. Pioneers in the world of sports, sleep and wellness are treating the female body as an undiscovered country, exploring it and understanding its idiosyncrasies. We can use that knowledge to flex our behaviours to perform, work and live better.

I used to periodically feel tired, overwhelmed by life and as if I was failing. Now, I try to flex my day to work with my 'hummingbird'/'owl' chronotype. I am more conscious of my menstrual cycle and try to schedule big events to avoid my 'Autumn' and coincide with my 'Summer'. It doesn't work all the time, as sometimes it's impossible to flex my calendar. But by trying, I feel more in control and no longer on the back foot. It has been a revelation. I'm kinder to myself, I respect my moods and my boundaries and, for me, it's a more sustainable way to live.

KATE SHEPHERD COHEN'S FLEX STORY

⊰⊰≻ ≺⊱⊱

*Kate Shepherd Cohen is a menstrual coach
and educator*

My period was never 'my' time of the month at all. It belonged to everyone else, just like every other day: friends and family and their needs; community and consumerism and its needs. It was a continuous sensation of being and feeling stuck in an outward-looking, ego-driven, high-energy motivational state: meetings every minute, late nights every night and alarms going off too early every morning. I began to suffer. Every two weeks, I felt deeply depressed and almost suicidal. It took me a long time to work out it was cyclical. I was diagnosed with PMDD [premenstrual dysphoric disorder] – severe PMT, which the doctor said was treatable through the contraceptive pill and antidepressants. My cycle was seen as an illness and a disorder.

I realized how little I knew about the menstrual cycle. I thought back to my biology lessons at school and vaguely remembered the diagram of the uterus and its thickening lining being shed. That's where my knowledge ended. How could this be, after 25 years of menstruation? Three hundred five-day periods! That's roughly 1,500 days of my life thought of, at best, as an inconvenience. My menstrual mission began in that moment. I swore to live by the natural rhythms of my own cycle, to harness the changing energies of my menstrual cycle. I soon discovered the work of menstrual godmothers Lucy H. Pearce, Alexandra Pope and Sjanie Hugo Wurlizer (founders of the Red School), and Miranda Gray, among others.

From not knowing where I was in my cycle and it wreaking havoc, it's now a central part of my life and supports me in everything we do as a family, to the point of proudly having my menstrual clock (with the hand pointing to the day of my cycle) hanging in our kitchen.

This clock is divided into quarters, showing the four seasons of my cycle, and lets the whole family know where I am. My husband loves it – he sees it as a roadmap to understand me. He can see where I am – for example, if I was overly critical he wouldn't take that personally. The clock gives me boundaries. In autumn I don't take on any new projects. I think about winter approaching and I would start to say no to socializing. It is significant to have the clock in the kitchen, in a public place, not in a shameful, hidden one. Women are at the heart of families; if our natural cycles are respected, everyone benefits.

The positive ripple effect of this cyclical self-care is enormous. It makes perfect sense that following deep rest for three days, I'm recharged and ready for the remainder of the month, able to be the best person I can be and of greater service to others. Living in harmony with the menstrual cycle (and being supported to do so), I believe, is the key to true feminine liberation.

'Step out of the
history that is holding
you back. Step into
the new story you are
willing to create.'

OPRAH WINFREY

FLEX

~

YOUR

~

FUTURE

When I was little, all adults asked children the same question. 'What do you want to be when you grow up?' Kids were trained to answer this. We picked something and stuck to it. I wanted to be a vet. My best friend Katie wanted to be an astronaut. Another kid – and this begs its own set of questions – wanted to be Pretty Woman. The idea was, as children, we were not yet our true selves. At some point we'd be 'grown up' and, at that moment, our identity would crystalize. The floaty bits of us would snap into focus and we'd solidify into the person we were meant to be. And we'd stay that same self. Our careers would be our identities. I would be a vet. Vet-ness would run through me like a stick of rock.

I'm not a vet. The closest I ever came to being one was having a dog. The question was flawed from the start. Adults still ask it, but I've noticed that children tend to answer 'I don't know' these days. My daughter tells me she thinks it's a stupid question. 'It changes all the time, Mummy. How can we know?'

She's right – how can we know? Independent forecaster Institute for the Future predicted that almost half of today's jobs may be replaced by automation in the next 20 years.[38]

85 per cent of the
jobs that will exist in
2030 haven't even
been invented yet.

Some jobs, like accountants, shop cashiers, call centre operators, bank tellers and pharmacists, may become extinct. And 85 per cent of the jobs that will exist in 2030 haven't even been invented yet. Who knows what these might be? Drone traffic controllers? End-of-life coaches? Telesurgeons? Techno-ethicists? Asking children to nail their ambitions down to a job that may no longer exist is nonsensical.

None of us can plan our lives forensically and rationally. There is no perfect route forward, with all the stars aligned. We don't know what's coming – maybe we never have, but now we really don't.

Globally, lifespans are increasing, our working lives are getting longer and we're facing a multitude of transitions – in love, in jobs, in life – along the way. This uncertainty opens up a whole new way of seeing life. This is not a time for definitive, rigid ten-year plans. It's a time for continual education, skilling and reskilling, side-hustling and career pivots – all of which require flexibility to adapt to new circumstances. It's a time, as Oprah said, to, 'Step into the new story you're willing to create.'

In this chapter, I will look at what longer life spans, new life paths and the march of artificial intelligence mean for the way we live and work. I'll look at how we can listen to our intuition and make decisions that pivot us in new directions. And I'll explore why flex is so important to future-proof ourselves, and live happy, fulfilled, long lives.

PLOT TWIST!
LETTING GO OF LIFE STAGES

No one knows the amount of time each of us has left on the earth. What is undeniable is that we are living longer. In the 1840s, British people lived, on average, until they were 40. That's my age as I write this. Today, more than one in four children born in the UK can expect to reach 100. In France, it is one in two.

With these longer lives stretching out ahead of us, blocks of time associated with distinct life stages are swapping and muddling together. Older people are going back to school and retraining. Younger people are leapfrogging higher education and becoming entrepreneurs. Marriage and children are delayed, or outright rejected. People of different ages and levels of experience will be studying, working, socializing together.

What is clear is that life is no longer a three-act play with a distinct beginning, middle and end. It doesn't start with education, continue with work and end with retirement. Rather, it's a collage of time-hops and plot twists; a mish-mash of experimentation and adaptation. So we need to let go of rigid assumptions of what young adulthood, midlife and older age are about.

Careers, today, are not for life. Today's learners will have eight to ten jobs by the time they are 38. This trend has been termed the 'quitting economy', and it involves switching between jobs as a way to get higher wages, accumulate experience and contacts, and avoid

THE RISE OF THE SIDE HUSTLE

According to a recent report called 'The Side Hustle Economy', as many as one in four adults are side-hustling, and these hustles generate income worth £72 billion for the UK. Emma Gannon, author of *The Multi-Hyphen Method*, says it is working for her: 'The ability to have more flexible working, to work on my own side projects, add different themes and strands to my work and personal identity . . . have all added to my own personal definition of success.'[39]

the stagnation of a fixed path. Quitting is no longer 'for losers'; it is a shrewd way to get ahead, to continually reinvent and re-sell yourself.

This capacity for reinvention is also expressed in the rise of side projects. These have been termed 'side hustles', and are usually defined as a small business or supplementary job on top of a main career to boost income, fulfil a passion or both.

Some worry about this more flexible approach to working, and blame it on a generational lack of loyalty. They say young people are always looking for something new, always obsessed with whether they feel 'fulfilled'. But this is to misunderstand the game. It's not just out of choice. They are quitting and switching jobs and side-hustling because they have to.

Today's young people are at risk of being the first generation since the Second World War to earn less than their parents. It is the precariousness of this changing world which forces young people to adapt and shape shift in order to keep on the front foot. Without the safety net and economic buoyancy of their parents' generation, they have to flex. And these skills will become more and more crucial for them as they age and the job market continually changes shape.

THE DECLINE OF 'ADULT' MILESTONES

The ultimate symbol of settling down, home ownership, is out of reach for the majority today. It is declining globally, as house prices are rising in every major city, and incomes are not keeping up. A 2017 report published by estate agents Knight Frank predicted that almost one in four households in Britain will be renting privately by the end of 2021 because of unaffordable house prices and stagnant wages.[40]

Numbers of child-free adults are on the rise. Figures show that nearly one in five women in England and Wales in their late forties have no children – compared to one in ten of their mother's generation.[41]

As people approach their forties, the markers of adulthood their parents bought into are becoming fainter and fainter. People aren't following the traditional grown-up script as much any more – buying property, getting married, having children. They complain about having to 'do adulting'. Badges of rebellion that used to signify youth are now the preserve of the middle-aged. A survey suggested that almost a quarter of 40- to 59-year-olds have a tattoo somewhere on their body, compared with under one in six of 18- to 24-year-olds. They don't want to grow up and settle down, and even if they did, they can't afford to.

So midlife is no longer about 'settling down'. And older age is not about slowing down, either.

My dad is 81, an accountant, and works a four-day week. My mum is running a café at 76. Both of them are relentless hard workers. Neither of them believe in

~~~~~~~~~~~~~~~~~~~~~~~~~~~~~~~

RETHINKING RETIREMENT

In the UK in 1948, the basic state pension age was 65 for men and 60 for women. Which made sense; at the time, life expectancy was 66 for men and 70 for women.

Life expectancy is so much higher today and pension costs are spiralling. The UK government is increasing the age at which you can claim a state pension to 66 from 2020, and the plan is to raise it to 67 by 2028. In addition to this, ONS figures show that since 1992, the number of people working beyond 64 years of age in the UK has doubled, and more than half of people aged 70 and over who are still working are self-employed.[42]

retirement, which they equate with cardigans, golf and the slow path to death. They barely believe in weekends. They are part of the zeitgeist. Today, the retirement age is increasing, people are working for longer and they don't appear to be slowing down.

Boomers who have paid off their mortgages and have decent pensions want to spend their money on experiences, for example travelling internationally and going on adventure holidays. And it's not just leisure – they are starting businesses too.

They are also divorcing, finding love in later life and staying sexually active. In fact, incidents of sexually transmitted infections amongst the over sixties have increased – so much so that PornHub, the online pornography platform, has released a sex-ed campaign aimed at the elderly (and they are giving away VHS copies to those who are less internet savvy).

Believe the stats and you paint a picture of a 70-year-old sexually active entrepreneur with wanderlust. Not someone playing golf in a cardigan.

So these are the demographic and cultural changes that are flexing our lifepaths. At the same time, the march of technology is creating new futures: of work, of education, of how we live our lives.

ARTIFICIAL INTELLIGENCE & WHAT IT *REALLY* MEANS TO BE HUMAN

The World Economic Forum calls today's technological changes the 'Fourth Industrial Revolution': life-changing breakthroughs in artificial intelligence, robotics, autonomous vehicles and 3-D printing.

These are incredible leaps forward, and will improve our lives in so many ways, yet they make us uneasy. A deep anxiety of our time is whether artificial intelligence will not only take our jobs but also make us redundant as humans.

In 2018, Sundar Pichai, CEO of Google, got up in front of the company's annual developer conference, held in Mountain View, California. Live on stage, he demonstrated how their artificial intelligence system, Google Assistant, could book a haircut. The tech community was blown away. It wasn't the task itself; we expect AI to start shouldering some of our dull, everyday tasks. What was jaw dropping was how the Google Assistant did it. The bot made a phone call to the hair salon, with a voice pattern so human, complete with 'mmhmms', pauses and chitchat, that the receptionist at the salon had no idea she was talking to a robot. If she had, would she have questioned whether that robot was coming after her own job?

For some of us, it might be sooner rather than later.

Google's Ray Kurzweil – a man Bill Gates calls 'the best person I know at predicting the future of artificial intelligence' – believes that humans will be outpaced by machines in 2029. That is, in 2029 the first computer will pass the Turing test, where the intelligence of the computer is indistinguishable from that of a human. By then, it is expected that artificial intelligence machines will be part of a company's board of directors. Perhaps it's most sensible to think of AI as our future co-worker: so, how will we work alongside it? How can we complement each other? What specific skills will we – as humans – bring to the party?

That last question is the killer. We need to reflect harder on what we humans are for, and what we are good at.

I believe one of the most urgent questions for my daughters' generation is not 'What do you want to be when your grow up?' but 'What is it, *really*, to be human today?'

In the workplace, we are rewarded for being able to perform like machines – long hours, productivity, efficiency. And this has leaked over into our private lives. We have allowed technology to chip away at the things which matter most to us. Sherry Turkle, clinical psychologist and sociologist at the Massachusetts Institute of Technology, worries how much we are voluntarily sacrificing at the altar of tech. She has shown that the mere presence of an iPhone on the table between two people makes them feel less connected and reduces the quality of their conversation. Even if it's turned face down. We will have a more shallow conversation, we will skirt over the things that matter, we will fail to look each other in the eyes, empathize and connect. It's as though the device looms large, still controlling us, a black hole of distraction and intimacy, even as it sits innocently with its back to us. Turkle believes that conversation, that most human of pastimes, is becoming endangered.

What is it, *really*, to be human today?

My phone already creates stock responses to emails I receive. If someone sends me an article, the phone offers me 'Thanks, I'll check it out' or 'Looks great!' as possible replies. Can you imagine if I succumbed and hit send and the person on the other end replied with the stock phrases her phone threw out? Our devices would be stuck in a loop of phatic, emotionless, nonsense conversations. It would be funny if it wasn't so depressing.

At the very point we should be nurturing our humanity as the thing that distinguishes us from AI, we are shedding it.

Bots are becoming more human-ish, and humans are becoming more robotic. It makes me think of the ending of George Orwell's *Animal Farm:* 'The creatures outside looked from pig to man, and from man to pig, and from pig to man again; but already it was impossible to say which was which.'

We're in a crucial moment in time. The pace of change is scorchingly fast compared to the past. Instead of racing to keep up, are we making the time to adjust, contemplate and be more intentional about our relationship with technology? Technology creeps up on us and makes itself at home, but we need to ask ourselves if it's really welcome.

HOW TO BE HUMAN IN A TECH-DRIVEN WORLD

~

Step away from your phone at key points in your day. There are whole books dedicated to helping us manage our relationship with technology addiction, but these are the things that have worked for me:

~ Don't charge your phone in your bedroom. Charge it in another room and buy an alarm clock.

~ Don't check your emails within an hour of waking up – otherwise you start the day responding to someone else's agenda rather than your own.

~ Put your phone in another room when you are with your family. A parent staring at their phone as a child tries to get eye contact is a common scenario. Try your hardest to avoid it.

Speak honestly and from the heart and avoid using buzzwords, jargon or stock phrases spewed out by your device. Many thanks!

Meet people face to face. Chat, look them in the eye, listen; don't just talk at people. Form rapport.

Be generous. Share ideas, do favours, introduce people.

HOW TO FLEX
YOUR FUTURE

So what should we be doing? With longer working lives, uncertain life paths and the unsettling rise of AI, the only thing we can be sure of is that we will need to flex, adapt and cope with change. What skills should we develop for more fulfilled, longer-lasting working lives?

1. Learn *how* to learn

For so long we've seen education as what we learn. A drip feed of information from teacher brain to student brain. Rote learning and testing happen along the way to check the info transaction is working. At some point, we take our info-full brains to the workplace and start spending this knowledge in return for money.

Except this doesn't work. The information kids get today floods them from all directions, not just from their teachers' brains. We need to teach them to interrogate the information they receive, to look at it critically. We need 'Post Truth' lessons in school. This will help children make sense of many conflicting shards of information, determine what to trust and what to dismiss, to find diverse voices rather than merely listening to the status quo, and to use this jigsaw to create a knowledgeable view on a topic.

But it's not just about turning a deluge of information into knowledge. We need to stop simply thinking about *what* we learn and start paying more attention to *how* we learn. In other words, help our kids re-learn how to learn. The knowledge they get from school and higher education will not be timeless and resilient to the pace of economic change – especially when the jobs we're training them for may not exist.

In the future, our ability to learn will be valued higher than what we already know. Our children need to leave school with the tools for 'learning in the moment' that they can use again and again as they pivot and flex through their careers.

This is the skill of coping with change, of being able to learn new things and leave old assumptions behind.

As Heather E. McGowan, an expert in the future of work, put it: 'Having an agile learning mind-set will be the new skill set of the twenty-first century.'[43]

2. **Check in with yourself every seven years**
A lifespan of 100 years is daunting and overwhelming. Avivah Wittenberg-Cox, gender expert and author of *Late Love: Mating in Maturity*, recommends breaking it down into seven-year blocks. Every seven years the body replaces itself with a largely new set of cells. Supposedly, the seven-year itch arrives in relationships. At the end of each block, we should take time out to contemplate, assess and plan (ideally with friends who are going through the same transitions – see point four on page 168).

You might ask yourself the following questions:

~ What have I learnt from the last seven years?
~ Do I still value the same things?
~ What should I leave behind?
~ What do I need to learn next?
~ Do I want to pivot and change something?

I found these questions really useful when we launched Starling. Adam and I wanted to leave behind the idea of business growth as aggressive targets and hiring more and more people. We wanted to think differently: growth with purpose, horizontal growth that stretched our boundaries, growth in our relationships with our clients.

I wanted to pivot towards a work life characterized by generosity – of time, ideas and conversations. And generosity with our colleagues to make sure we all had whatever we needed to work best and happiest – and very often this is flexibility.

It really helped to be intentional about this when we started our business. As Wittenberg-Cox says: 'You figure out life in the rearview mirror – it doesn't make sense when you are actually going through it. Why do we tend to take the time to contemplate when it's too late? Better to do it earlier.'

Some of this involves getting to grips with how to leave behind what is no longer right, useful or relevant. Like a snake shedding the skin that no longer fits, we need to identify and shed the skills, practices and opinions which no longer serve us.

3. **Reskill, pivot, side-hustle**

As a result of this introspection, we'll see people deciding to pivot their careers, go back to education or start side-hustles. This is a difficult choice, no matter how much soul-searching you have done. It's hard to move on from a stable job; it's unnerving to swap directions. It's especially difficult for older people – the adult brain is less flexible than the teenage brain, which is primed for change and novelty.

So how can we navigate our own reinvention? One way is to borrow from the Japanese concept of *Ikigai* or 'a reason for being'. The model, designed in a beautiful intersecting diagram, asks the following four questions:

~ What do I love?
~ What am I good at?
~ What can I be paid for now? (Or could this become a future side-hustle?)
~ What does the world need?

It's a useful set of questions to help us work out what we really value in our lives, where our skills lie and what we want to prioritize going forwards. It can help us decide where to pivot or what hustle to pursue.

Writing this book is my side-hustle. I'm good at coming up with ideas. I love writing. I believe the world needs flex. *Ikigai* would tell me to go for it.

As a result of all this introspection, we'll see older people going back to education and taking undergraduate degrees, or retraining in new industries and starting at the bottom rung again.

A great example of this is Now Teach, a scheme set up by former *Financial Times* journalist Lucy Kellaway, which targets disillusioned and burnt-out professionals approaching retirement age and helps them to pivot into teaching.

'For me, this had been a long time coming,' she says. 'When my mum died I thought I'd had it with journalism because it was too shallow . . . I was sat around with all these journalists fussing over what the headline was, and I thought: "No, I don't want to do this any more. I want to do something useful."'

TIMOTHY PHILLIPS' FLEX STORY

*Timothy Phillips is an author and works for
a government spending watchdog*

It finally happened one afternoon in 2010 when I was on holiday at the seaside. Sitting in a pub garden, discussing how I felt with some of my best friends, I suddenly felt the balance tip and I knew that when I returned to London I would definitely be applying to go part-time at my salaried job in order to create proper space to pursue my other interest, writing.

I was already a published author, but now, midway through my second book, I had ended up with greatly increased responsibilities in my salaried job, meaning that it was a real struggle to fit everything else in.

I am well aware that, faced with this problem, not everyone can afford to opt for the salary cut. I was very fortunate to be in that position. But, even so, I found that I had to overcome powerful stigmas, both social and personal, in order to take the part-time route.

Might I be sidelined in future considerations for promotion, I worried. Wasn't I opting to enter a cul-de-sac in career terms, and thereby signalling a lack of ambition and, more fundamentally, a lack of clarity in my life? Rather than focusing on doing one thing well, didn't I run the risk of doing two things badly?

In that pub garden, I suddenly realized that I owed it to myself to give the twin careers approach a try. After all, I was genuinely enjoying both my jobs and I knew that each of them satisfied different needs and provided me with fulfilment in different ways.

I am glad to say that I have never regretted my decision. My second book was published in 2017 and I am now planning a third. I got back some of the free time I had previously lost through being too busy and have used it to do the things that people need to do in order to relax and recuperate: to enjoy my family, to exercise, to read for pleasure.

Even in the part of my life where I was prepared to take a hit, I have been surprised to find that my bosses have not overlooked me for promotion, and also that they have respected my contracted hours. As so many professionals who go part-time say, I have definitely learned to work more efficiently than in the past and I now find it easier to be decisive in the workplace and to empower my teams through delegation and by trusting them more.

I think I originally suspected that, someday, one of my two careers would end up taking the lead again and that I would leave the other one behind. But now I'm not so sure. I feel that the two together help me to achieve an equilibrium in my life in a way that neither on its own could supply.'

So Kellaway set up Now Teach for older people who want to spend their energy and time doing something meaningful. One thousand people applied and were whittled down to the first cohort of 45. Kellaway is now a maths teacher in east London, and finds it 'exhilarating, alien, exciting, exhausting. I'm mentally pinching myself every minute of the day thinking, "Am I really a teacher?"'[44]

4. **Love your friends**
We are living longer and going through more ups, downs and transitions along the way. We can share some of our emotional decision-making with partners and family members, but it's still a lot to take on. We need friendships more than ever to sustain and inspire us. Long-running studies have shown that people who have quality, warm friendships in their lives are healthier, happier and live longer.

We have neglected our friends, though. Philosopher Alain de Botton wrote: 'A good set of friends can be the making of a really good life. But it's just very, very hard to find. We are obsessed by our careers and by our love life. Friendships come very much third, particularly when people start to have children – friends really go out the window then.'[45]

THE GLOBAL LONELINESS EPIDEMIC

According to the Office for National Statistics, in 2016 to 2017, 5 per cent of people over 16 – or 1 in 20 adults – in England report feeling lonely often or always.[46] According to a 2018 Ipsos survey of 20,000 US adults, nearly half of Americans report sometimes or always feeling alone or left out.[47]

In South Korea, single-person households constitute more than a quarter of all households in the country. Loneliness in South Korea has even spawned a new subculture called *honjok* – a term which loosely means 'loners', combining 'hon' (alone) and 'jok' (tribe).

We need friends, but we've forgotten how to do friendship.

Okinawa in Japan is one of the world's 'Blue Zones' (regions of the world where people live much longer than average). There, people form a social network called a *moai*. Traditionally, when a child is born, they are put into a group with four other children born around the same time. This is their *moai*, a lifelong crew. Together they support each other –emotionally, socially, even financially – over a lifetime, meeting regularly to exchange news and gossip and offer advice.

I like the idea of the *moai*. But you can't just snap your fingers and get a ready-made *moai*. Studies say two people need to spend 90 hours together to become friends, or 200 hours to qualify as close friends. Clearly we need to invest time and energy in our friendships.

But how? Instead of digging into academic studies to determine the rules of sustaining enriching friendships, I decided to take my own advice and act more like a human. I asked my own friends. Here's what they said:

1. **Have interweaving lives.** Know and care about each other's friends and families. One friend is an advocate of the 'minestrone', a dinner party deliberately mixing people from different parts of your life into one big friend soup. She says this means your friendships deepen, because there are more cross-connections. But it also shows you for who you are in your entirety, rather than fragmenting yourself for different types of friends.

2. **Have shared experiences** (like weekends away, dinners, hanging out and watching Eurovision) rather than just snatched coffees to catch up on separate lives. A few friends criticize the 'catch-up coffee', saying it shouldn't be the only way you interact. It relies too much on the past and the frantic present. It doesn't invest you in the future of your relationship. Unlike point three . . .

3. **Have parties!** Parties make new stories and memories. They mark milestones, they celebrate being alive and they involve dancing. The best ones have conga lines.

4. **Ask for help**; don't just present a polished, Instagrammable, perfect life to each other. Help can be as small as asking a friend to do the school run, or as big as asking for support when you are going through a sad time. It doesn't just benefit you. People like being asked for help.

5. **But don't be a 'friend parasite'.** We all have that friend who habitually offloads their problems in energy-sapping monologues, without asking a single question in return. Each encounter with the 'friend parasite' leaves you feeling drained and a bit diminished.

6. **Be generous about changing circumstances.** Allow friendships to flex and evolve. Don't hold your friends hostage to the people they were when you met.

7. **Be kind.** Don't demand every meet-up is exciting and fun. Allow each other to be tired and fed up sometimes.

8. **Be tolerant.** Don't judge them too much, or hold them to impossible standards. A friend's grandpa always said: 'You've got to shut one eye to make a friend and both eyes to keep them.'

9. **Have a range of friends:** don't expect the world from any one person.

SUMMARY

My 81-year-old accountant dad hates computers.
It's clear the robots are coming for a big slice of his job.
Number crunching, analysis, spreadsheets – all of these
will be done by something like the Google Assistant
that was so good at booking a haircut.

But he has future-proofed himself because his clients
love him for his humanity, his empathy, his complex
problem-solving. These are exactly the qualities that
machines will never be able to rival. Listening to
someone going through a transition like divorce or
death of a loved one and helping them work out what
to do next is at heart of the human experience in these
changing times. Being a friend and having friends staves
off sadness and ill-health. The skills of friendship can
reduce the likelihood of a robot taking your job.

We need to be able to show sensitivity and compassion to
ourselves – whether it is every seven years, as advocated by
Wittenberg-Cox, or at regular points with our version of
a *moai*, throughout our increasingly zig-zagging journey
through life. This will help us pivot, adapt and evolve as
the world around us changes. Because the ability to flex to
change will be a super-power. As futurist and philosopher
Alvin Toffler said: 'The illiterate of the twenty-first
century will not be those who cannot read and write,
but those who cannot learn, unlearn and relearn.'

'Historically, pandemics have forced humans to break with the past and imagine their world anew. This one is no different. It is a portal, a gateway between one world and the next... we can walk through lightly, with little luggage, ready to imagine another world. And ready to fight for it.'

ARUNDHATI ROY

FLEX

~

IN

~

FLUX

What the F is flex in a Covid-19 world? Before the outbreak of Covid-19 in 2020, I had been researching and banging on about flex for 20 years. Chipping away at the barriers, the prejudice and the 'flexism' – the stagnancy of the status quo that repeated 'it can't work'. During that period, I worked in trends and futures for trailblazing brands. The reports I read, the experts I interviewed, the data I pored over, all of it told me that flex was an idea that had come of age.

My partner and I named our trends business Starling because if you've ever seen an actual starling murmuration, you'll have felt its magic and awe. Murmurations of starlings swirl above you in a collective dance, individual birds reacting to opportunities and threats, coming together into one breathtaking, powerful force.

The most wild, innovative and beautiful ideas are like murmurations. They have many elements which collide and coalesce to make change happen. Yet they move us with their simplicity and their potency. For years, flex was a wild idea, a starling murmuration in my head. I collected the cultural signals that were swooping above us and building momentum.

Signals such as:

~ The explosion of tech which connects us

~ Longer working days and the crisis of productivity

~ Burnout epidemic in workplaces worldwide

~ New ideals of success around personal growth

~ The beautiful, messy outlines of the modern family

~ The practice of self-optimization

~ The ageing population needing longer,
  sustainable careers

~ The global rise of women in the workplace

~ Women's second and third shifts, and the emotional
  load at home

~ The climate crisis which forces us to reassess our
  wasteful lifestyles

~ The glaring lack of diversity in today's workforce

Flex was an idea at the fringes that was surely set to tip over into the mainstream, I thought. I was right, but for the wrong reasons.

What I didn't factor in was a global pandemic. The shift towards flex didn't happen organically as the signals listed above reached maturity. The shift happened in a fear-fuelled rush, as we plunged into lockdown, forbidden to see friends and family, never mind colleagues. With home-working thrust upon us, and desperate to find a way to work through the crisis, companies that had long-insisted flexible working couldn't work were scrambling to make it a reality. The barriers melted away. The U-turns were dizzying. I watched the mass adoption of ideas that for years were criticised as leftfield, impractical and naïve.

I spoke at a pre-Covid event at which one business owner told me that flex would never work in his industry because clients needed 24/7 responsiveness. Months later, he rolled out his plan for part-time office hours to great applause and recognition of his empathetic leadership. Facebook expects half their future workforce will be permanently remote.[48] More traditional businesses have also committed to a flexible future. James Gorman, CEO of Morgan Stanley, said they had proved they can operate with 'effectively no footprint' and will have 'much less real estate' in the future.[49]

And employers' biggest fears about flexible working, that we would all 'shirk from home' and productivity would spiral, proved to be groundless. Among first-time flexers working at home during the lockdown, 68 per cent feel they are either more productive or equally productive.[50]

So, is flex the 'new normal'? Is our work here done? Well, no, no it's not. We need to scrutinize what it is exactly that we have experienced. And it's not flex. Flex isn't working from home during a pandemic. We've seen our homes turned into makeshift offices, schools and gyms. And while some have sat in the peace and comfort of a study, others have perched on the edges of beds with aching backs. Parents have attempted homeschooling while desperately trying to hang onto their jobs. We've worried and pined for our elders. We've caught the virus and got sick. We've felt cut off and lonely. Some have experienced domestic violence. We've coped with grief and anxiety, we've been made redundant. Covid-19 is a storm that everyone in the world has weathered. But each one of us has had a different boat – some had tankers and some barely had rafts. Covid is a leveller which has, at the same time, crystallized society's starkest inequalities.

This is not flexible working, it's an emergency which we've been dealing with as best we can. Flex as an ideology that has come of age is not what we've been experiencing. But we've learnt so much about what works, what doesn't, and the kinds of futures we want to create. Despite the crisis, there are green shoots of hope. Green shoots which are resilient and strong, yet bend as things change and new needs arise. This chapter is about those green shoots and what I believe is the future of flex in a post-pandemic age.

ZOOM DOOM & HARD EDGES

First of all, let's be honest about what hasn't worked. In our rush to work from home, we have made the mistake of allowing old toxic habits into our homes. A study by the US National Bureau of Economic Research shows the impact of lockdown: our already long working hours have lengthened. The average workday increased by 48 minutes after lockdown and the number of meetings rose by 13 per cent.[51] Microsoft's data agrees, suggesting lockdown has seen people working four more hours a week.[52]

We've swapped physical presenteeism for digital presenteeism. We've been given autonomy over our time and instead of embracing it for our own health and happiness, we have fallen into overwork and overwhelm. Pre-pandemic research confirms this: those with more flexibility and control over their time actually end up working longer hours not fewer. [53] Why would we do this? Partly because we're grateful for flex so we repay it with overwork. Partly because everything is that little bit harder and slower. In part because we feel insecure in these fraught times, so we show our commitment by getting trigger-happy with the reply button. But mostly because of a longer-term trend: the Great Blur between home and work caused by constant connectivity, open plan spaces and a culture that equates success with busyness. The Cult of Busy is hard to unpick. Studies show that the most successful people are perceived to be the busiest. [54] How many times have you asked someone how they are and been met with the 'Crazy busy!' swagger of the Very Important and Successful Human?

6

We've swapped physical presenteeism for digital presenteeism.

9

But trading the nine-to-five for the 24/7 is a massive fail. We need hard edges to our flex, particularly now, or we'll slip into the burnout from which we were hoping to escape. What can we do to reinstate boundaries? We need to savour our saved time. If we no longer have commutes, we can use that time for ourselves (exercising, reading, calling friends and family for a chat, shifting our days earlier or later to harmonize with circadian rhythms – see page 115, *Flex & the Body* chapter).

We can consciously do simple things like closing the laptop and going for a walk before coming back to work; or refusing to eat 'al desko' and ensuring we take a full lunch break. Or digitally intervening and putting time limits on social media. One friend capped her emails during lockdown so she could not send anything after 7pm. A norm I hope to see is the inclusion of details of our flex pattern as part of our email signature, citing what time we log off.

Boundaries are not solely the responsibility of the individual. We need our employers to create systems which discourage digital presenteeism. France's 'right to disconnect' is a measure to cut out-of-hours emailing. Advertising agencies like Digitas and Crispin Porter Bogusky have instituted 'protected time' free from meetings for all employees.

Once we have erected hard edges, the next step is to interrogate the ways we have been working. Post-lockdown, we sleepwalked into a Zoom culture, and it's draining us. Scared of being atomized and disconnected, we filled our days with video meetings. They are indeed a great way to share information, but they were not the elixir we'd hoped for.

Here are some of the issues: Video meetings are not relaxing. We're paralysed with fear that our kid / pet / naked husband is going to wander into shot. Someone always forgets to turn off the mute button. Anxiety-making time lags are filled with nervous chatter. We try to decode people's expressions; are they bored, frozen, both? And our own expressions start to haunt us. You know the way that, if you write the same word too many times, you start to mistrust your own spelling? The same thing happens on a Zoom call, but with your face. You become acutely aware of it. It starts to look odd. You experiment with different facial expressions to convey alert attentiveness. Performative engagement through the medium of smiles, nods and thumbs up. It's exhausting. And as research is beginning to show, Zoom fatigue is real. [55]

Not only that, it can amplify existing inequalities. A survey of remote employees found that 37 per cent believe that working remotely can lead to reduced visibility and less access to company leadership.[56] An online meeting space can give license to the same old voices dominating the agenda. If you have the backdrop of a nice home office, a partner dealing with the kids out of shot and zero worries about interruptions, it's easy for you to 'own the Zoom'.

Some of us turn off our cameras not because we're disengaged but because we have a whole load of stuff happening at home which we're not comfortable with sharing. Piles of laundry, kids having tantrums, worries that the place we call home will be sneered at and judged; all of this might make us mute ourselves, and shrink our professional impact at the same time.

Managers need to read the Zoom, notice who speaks, who is silent and who is invisible. An empathetic phone call to find out why is key. Progressive businesses don't default to digital meetings for every occasion. They use different communication options depending on the need – and are clear on when and how to use them. Workplace chat app Slack for knowledge sharing, phone calls for more direct conversations, a walk in the park to generate ideas and get on the same page, a webinar for training, emails with clear rules of engagement about urgency of response needed. Otherwise we fall into the trap of metabolizing work's existing toxicity, spewing it into the digital space, and pretending that it's flex.

THE GENDER PENALTY

One of the many catastrophic effects of Covid-19 has been its impact on women's careers. In the UK mothers were 47 per cent more likely to have permanently lost their job or quit, and 14 per cent were more likely to have been furloughed since the start of the crisis. [57] Flex and the Home is all about the emotional load falling disproportionately on women's shoulders and holding their careers back. Because without equity at home, there is little hope for it at work.

Lockdown turbo-charged this issue and propelled it onto the political stage. British campaign group Pregnant Then Screwed said working mothers are 'sacrificial lambs' in the coronavirus childcare crisis. In their research, of those who had been, or expected to be, made redundant, 46 per cent said lack of childcare played a role. [58] It's no wonder then that working mothers have been able to do only one hour of uninterrupted paid work for every three hours done by men during lockdown.

This lack of flow is something that I've experienced. Just today, I sat down to write this chapter. My youngest wanted to show me approximately seven magic tricks in a row. Then the dog was sick – twice – and I then had to pick my eldest up from a playdate. If only those magic tricks could conjure me some time. I'm not the only one. In the academic world, the number of article submissions from women dropped significantly at the start of lockdown, whereas those from men were up almost 50 per cent in the same month. [59]

Women are in danger of losing all the gains we have made. Sam Smethers, the chief executive of the Fawcett Society, says: 'It's taken us twenty years to get this far on female participation in the workforce, but it could take only months to unravel.'

So what to do? We must not let this period turn back the clock. Each and every one of us needs to talk about it. Negotiate with one another. Take turns with everything. Share the load.

Governments desperately need to solve the childcare crisis and get the schools working again. Business needs to acknowledge and assist mothers.

I'm interested in the idea of 'emotional load concierges' – how can employers help shoulder that burden and how will that impact the number of women reaching senior positions? I hope we'll see the take-up of parental leave (shockingly low at the moment [60]) rewarded, even identified as the reason for promotion.

And the money that businesses will save as they shrink their real estate will be rechannelled into equipping their workers with the right infrastructure at home to work comfortably. This will level the playing field between the haves and the have-nots. Domain name company Nominet began lockdown by shipping office chairs, monitors and keyboards to its staff. Google CEO Sundar Pichai announced plans for a $1,000 grant for each employee for home office equipment and furniture.

"

We must not let this
period turn back the
clock.

"

Another progressive move would be re-thinking 'perks'. The perks of the past were fridges full of free food, massages, ping pong, gyms, haircuts and dry cleaning on site. This is the perk as a 'stay-here' tactic, based on the assumption that presence means productivity. Perks had a centripetal force, they pulled us inwards towards the mothership.

But perks of the future may well be centrifugal, pushing us outwards and helping us with our lives outside the four walls of our workplaces. We could see complementary 'side-hustle mentorship', to encourage us to follow our passions as well as trusting us to do our jobs; in other words, treating us like grown-ups with broad ambitions rather than infantilizing us with pinball machines and bean bags.

And the elusive conjuring trick of women's time? I have been trying to hack the moments I have by wearing headphones and belting my eardrums with playlists which fast-track my concentration. Virginia Woolf said that a woman needs a room of her own to have the freedom to write and be creative. Find a room of your own, and by a room I mean a toilet seat, a spot on the stairs, an arm of the sofa – anywhere that gives you a smidgen of uninterrupted privacy. And think, work, concentrate and just be.

THE FUTURE OF THE OFFICE: TWATS, EGGS & CHAT ROULETTE

According to the newspapers, it is very binary: we'll either see the death of the office in a completely remote world or we will snap back to 'normal' as though nothing has happened. Neither seems likely. One thing is for sure, the default of full-time and the dominance of the office is over. It's already starting. In the UK, for the first time, part-time season train tickets are being introduced for flexi-workers.

The notion of us all getting on a train or bus at exactly the same time in synchronized, dense, unhygienic, stressful commutes at the beginning and end of each weekday will seem absurd. Yes, sometimes we will all want to be in the same place at the same time, but that won't necessarily be Monday to Friday, 9-to-5. People simply don't want it any more. A survey of 1,500 workers found that just 1 per cent wanted to return full-time to the office. Over half of employees wanted an 80 per cent virtual, 20 per cent office-based split. [61]

So the future of work is most likely to be hybrid – a blend of office and location-flex. We might shrink to four-day weeks. Or become TWaTs[62] (where we're only in the office on Tuesday, Wednesday and Thursday). I imagine there would be a more staggered start and end to the day, with agreed core hours in between.

This doesn't mean when we're not in the office, we'll all be working from home, which became the necessary assumption during the pandemic. It's undeniable that loneliness was a growing problem that was accentuated by Covid-19. Solo households, social distancing and continued working from home could cause acute widespread isolation. A solution would be the adoption of working near home (WNH).

These WNH neighbourhood hubs could incorporate spaces for co-working, local food stands, crèches, adult education with lifelong learning modules and spaces for different generations to socialize and look out for each other. This is a far cry from the millennial-obsessed, flat-white-chugging co-working spaces that have sprung up in the city centres. One thing we have been experiencing during lockdown is more community in neighbourhoods, more connection to our local food suppliers, burgeoning friendships with our neighbours no matter their age. WNH spaces will allow that social glue to prevail – with genuine inclusion at the heart – with hubs for everyone, where everyone is welcome.

This, in turn, will influence the make-up of the modern city. Architect Cedric Price came up with the analogy of the city as an egg.[63] Over time, the type of egg has evolved. In ancient times it resembled a boiled egg – with the dense centre protected by the shell of the city walls. It then evolved to the fried egg model – the yolk as the financial centre and the white as the ever-expanding suburbs, as cities grew outwards. In fact, it was fears about disease and air pollution in the nineteenth and early twentieth centuries which spurred the exodus from city centres and the suburban spread. Sound familiar?

The next iteration is the scrambled egg city, powered by a new wave of counter-urbanization as people yearn for more space for their money – for home offices and gardens. The scrambled egg is where our WNH hubs are dispersed throughout the suburbs and scrambled together with our residential districts. Inner city skyscraper office blocks will lose their status. Like vertical cruise ships, no open windows and long queues for elevators, they will seem risky, even icky. They'll need to become contact-less; in which case the hallways will echo with requests for Alexa to open doors for us and make us a coffee.

Despite all of this, the centralized workplace won't die. Our time within it will be much more intentional. Solo, silo-ed work, where workers wore headphones at hotdesks, tapping away in silence next to each other will seem bananas. If you want to do deep-focused, solo work, why brave the commute and the cruise ship, I mean the office, at all?

Now, when we do come into the office, we will want specifically designed collaborative spaces intended to create conversations. The amount of desk space would shrink to make way for creative interactive spaces. We will want modular furniture that can be repurposed and adapted depending on who is in and what they need to achieve. Biophilic offices, where greenery infuses our spaces, will keep us connected to nature. We will need places of empathy where we can read one another, feel belonging and cohesion, build teams and plan together.

If you want to do deep focused, solo work, why brave the commute and the office at all?

But there can't be too much deliberation in our work at the expense of chance. If all our work together is purposeful and planned, what about those serendipitous conversations which happen as you wait for a lift or make tea? In traditional full-time offices, you often bump into someone you wouldn't normally speak to – so-called 'weak ties'.[64] You might have conversations over that clichéd watercooler, find common ground and circulate ideas. That is where the magic happens, isn't it? Steve Jobs designed Pixar Animation Studios in California[65] to increase the chance of inadvertent encounters. It has a large, central, multi-purpose atrium which houses everything from the restaurant to the meeting rooms, the mailboxes to the bathrooms. Employees across the studios need to criss-cross through this space multiple times a day. Said Jobs: 'You stumble across someone, ask what he's up to, are surprised, and suddenly everything is seething with possible ideas.'[66] The potential for magic collisions is immeasurable.

If we are working more flexibly and with less physical proximity how can we inject some of that serendipity into our lives? How can we build relationships with new people and not just solidify old ones? This is called the 'propinquity effect': the tendency to develop deeper relationships with those we see most regularly, who, for example, sit next to us at work, or those in our direct teams who we speak to regularly on Zoom meetings.

My answer is a digital one. Readers of a certain age might remember Chatroulette, a chatroom in the early 2000s that paired random users for webcam-based conversations. You could end up speaking to anyone, anywhere in the world. When the conversation dried up, you clicked 'next' and you would be taken to a new chat with another randomly selected person. Some of these encounters were inspiring; I remember a woman in Lithuania excitedly telling me all about her new restaurant opening. And some were less so – the website was plagued with men flashing their private parts. Yet the premise was a good one: digital serendipity by design.

A similar concept for work might be the way forward, with colleagues you normally wouldn't speak to or 'bump into' in the average working day. This would encourage a flow of ideas and would not be reliant on physical proximity or existing relationships. Maybe every Thursday we reserve an hour slot for Work Roulette, where we are paired with random colleagues, with no agenda other than conversation. We could measure the subsequent cross-pollinated projects and resulting innovation. All the magic of serendipity, just with fewer flashers.

WHAT NOW?

Remote working in a pandemic has the potential to be so much more than the emergency response to a crisis. Just as flex itself is so much more than the flexible working request on paper. It's deeper than the logistics of how, where and when we work. There's always a profoundly human story behind the request. And that brought me to the topic in the first place. Flex is the passion of a new business idea, the parent with dementia, the desire to write a novel, the diagnosis of a disability. It's birth, death, hope and fear. The end of one chapter and the start of the next. The diversity of these stories hold one thing in common – their power to trigger our empathy.

As economic and social recovery progresses, lots of new models for flex will arise. We will experiment; we will try out new templates because the notion of flex is in itself flexible. But we'll always know that what we share is more powerful than our different patterns of living and working. Novelist Henry James said: 'Three things in human life are important: the first is to be kind; the second is to be kind; and the third is to be kind.' As long as we're listening, as long as we're kind, we'll keep flexing.

'The illiterate of the twenty-first century will not be those who cannot read and write, but those who cannot learn, unlearn and relearn.'

ALVIN TOFFLER

AFTER
WORD

I n this book, I've looked at flex across different areas of our lives – creativity and flexibility of thinking; work and the nine-to-five; home, relationships and the emotional load; our body and its rhythms and cycles; and our futures.

Thinking flexibly in all of these areas has changed my life. But it hasn't always been easy. There was the three-day working week which turned into a shitshow; the years of tiredness and forcing myself to be productive before I understood my body's rhythms and cycles; the endless meetings and screen-time which stifled creative thought. Since I have learned how to flex, I have found the confidence to face up to challenges and apparent impasses with a bravery and inventiveness I couldn't have mustered before.

At first glance, the word 'flexibility' may appear to describe something that is soft or pliable. Flexible people might seem like pushovers, bending over backwards to fit in, marching to someone else's drum. But I hope I have shown here that flex gives us power; to flex is to show immense strength.

It does not mean succumbing to the ever-increasing demands on our time and attention. Done right, on our own terms, it gives us resilience to our toxic culture of presenteeism, time-pressure and ultimately burnout.

It helps us escape the army of octopus lady jugglers, crazed with the exhaustion of 'having it all'. It allows us to live longer lives more sustainably. It gives us self-worth – which brings with it the ability to say no when something doesn't work for us, and yes when it does. And as much as we want to own our own time, we don't want to do all of this alone. We want to work out how to flex with the people who are most precious to us.

Flex doesn't mean messy. When done right, flex has sharp edges. Flex embodies the definitive decisions we make when circumstances change, and the precise limits of our own energy and capacity. It is the boundaries we put in place to protect us, such as new lines drawn in the home to share the load and share the joy. Flex is the space we make for our own creativity, which intensifies it and makes it thrive and flourish.

Flex is brave. It takes chutzpah to challenge society's norms and the structures that surround us. To break our way out of echo chambers. To call out what's wrong and invent new solutions. Perhaps the bravest thing of all is not knowing all the answers, but having the courage to experiment, to invent, to make things up as we go.

Because, when you boil it all down, flex is about asking ourselves one big question: How do I want to live this beautiful life? And then going out there and doing it.

REFERENCES

1 Rothman, Joshua, 'Creativity Creep', *New Yorker*, 2 September 2014

2 Asimov, Isaac, 'On Creativity', *Technology Review*, January/February 2015

3 From a study conducted by researchers at the University of California, San Diego, see www.nytimes.com/2009/12/10/technology/10data.html

4 'The Cost of Interrupted Work: More Speed and Stress', 2008, www.ics.uci.edu/~gmark/chi08-mark.pdf

5 Tadmor, Carmit T. *et al.*, 'Not Just for Stereotyping Anymore: Racial Essentialism Reduces Domain-General Creativity', *Psychological Science*, Vol. 24, Iss. 1, January 2013

6 See blog.ted.com/walking-meetings-5-surprising-thinkers-who-swore-by-them/

7 'Give Your Ideas Some Legs: The Positive Effect of Walking on Creative Thinking', 2014, www.apa.org/pubs/journals/releases/xlm-a0036577.pdf

8 'Interview: Jerry Seinfeld on how to be funny without sex and swearing' 5 Jan 2014, www.theguardian.com/culture/2014/jan/05/jerry-seinfeld-funny-sex-swearing-sitcom-comedy

9 Dave Chappelle to Jerry Seinfeld, *Comedians in Cars Getting Coffee* Season 10, July 2018

10 'International comparisons of UK productivity (ICP), final estimates: 2015', 5 April 2017, www.ons.gov.uk/economy/economicoutputandproductivity/productivitymeasures/bulletins/internationalcomparisonsofproductivity finalestimates/2015

11 'Presenteeism hits record high in UK organisations as stress at work rises', May 2018, www.cipd.co.uk/about/media/press/020518-health-wellbeing-survey

12 'Employees spend 2.5 weeks a year working when ill – costing businesses £4k per employee in lost productivity', October 2017, www.ntu.ac.uk/about-us/news/news-articles/2017/10/employees-spend-2.5-weeks-a-year-working-when-ill-costing-businesses-4k-per-employee-in-lost-productivity

13 'CIPD Health and Well-being at Work Report – 2018', www.insights.simplyhealth.co.uk/insights/cipd-health-and-well-being-at-work-report-2018

14 From a poll of 2,000 adults undertaken as part of research by the charity Mental Health UK, d1wk4hs734fd0n.cloudfront.net/assets/genesis/landing_pages/MHAW/eve_mattress_infographic_final.png

15 'The Future is Flexible: The Importance of Flexibility in the Modern Workplace', www.werk.co/research

16 'Salary Survey 2018: Wellbeing and the future of work', 11 January 2018, www.marketingweek.com/2018/01/11/salary-survey-2018-wellbeing-and-the-future-of-work/

17 'Five Facts About Family Caregivers', 15 November 2015, www.pewresearch.org/fact-tank/2015/11/18/5-facts-about-family-caregivers/

18 'Flexible working provision and uptake', May 2012, www.ask4flex.org/UK-_Flexible_Working_Survey_Report--CIPD.pdf

19 'The Future is Flexible: The Importance of Flexibility in the Modern Workplace', werk.co/documents/The%20Future%20is%20Flexible%20-%20Werk%20Flexibility%20Study.pdf

20 'Why Working from Home Is a "Future-looking Technology"', 22 June 2017, www.gsb.stanford.edu/insights/why-working-home-future-looking-technology

21 'Deloitte Survey: Less Than Half of People Surveyed Feel Their Organization Helps Men Feel Comfortable Taking Parental Leave', 15 June 2016, www.prnewswire.com/news-releases/deloitte-survey-less-than-half-of-people-surveyed-feel-their-organization-helps-men-feel-comfortable-taking-parental-leave-300284822.html

22 'The plan to ban work emails out of hours', www.bbc.co.uk/news/magazine-36249647, 11 May 2016

23 Slaughter, Anne-Marie, 'Why Women Still Can't Have It All', *Atlantic*, July/August 2012

24 'Working Women: Key facts and trends in female labor force participation', 16 October 2017, www.ourworldindata.org/female-labor-force-participation-key-facts

25 'Women shoulder the responsibility of "unpaid work"', 10 November 2016, www.ons.gov.uk/employment andlabourmarket/peopleinwork/earningsandworkinghours/articles womenshouldertheresponsibility ofunpaidwork/2016-11-10

26 Westervelt, Amy, 'In Japan, the rise of the house husband redraws established gender norms' *Post Magazine*, July 2018

27 Rhodes, Giulia, '"It was like a marriage, only better": the single mothers who moved in together', *Guardian*, 29 September 2018

28 Bauman, Valerie, 'Chore wars: American men are helping out more around the house – but women aren't doing any less work as a result, data says', dailymail.com, 15 August 2018

29 Khazan, Olga, 'Emasculated Men Refuse to Do Chores – Except Cooking', *Atlantic*, 24 October 2016

30 'Not All Housework is Created Equal: Particular Housework Tasks and Couples' Relationship Quality', 3 April 2016 www.contemporaryfamilies.org/houseworkandrelationshipquality/

31 'Men enjoy five hours more leisure time per week than women', 9 January 2018, www.ons.gov.uk/peoplepopulation andcommunity/wellbeing/articles/men enjoyfivehoursmore leisuretimeperweek thanwomen/2018-01-09

32 Brewer, Gayle and Hendrie, Colin A., 'Evidence to suggest that copulatory vocalizations in women are not a reflexive consequence of orgasm', *Archives of Sexual Behavior*, Vol. 40, Iss. 3, June 2011

33 'Mumsnet's Justine Roberts: I made a list of all our jobs on a spreadsheet. I had 65 and my husband had five', 30 May 2013, www.standard.co.uk/lifestyle/london-life/mumsnets-justine-roberts-i-made-a-list-of-all-our-jobs-on-a-spreadsheet-i-had-65-and-my-husband-had-8637312

34 'Same- and Different-Sex Couples Negotiating at Home', www.familiesand work.org/downloads/modern-families.pdf

35 Read, Erin, 'Whether a Husband Identifies as a Breadwinner Depends on Whether He Respects His Wife's Career – Not on How Much She Earns', *Harvard Business Review*, 15 August 2018

36 See www.sleepfoundation.org/sleep-topics/teens-and-sleep

37 See Lyttleton, Ben, *Edge: Leadership secrets from Football's Top Thinkers*, HarperCollins, 2017.

38 'The Future of Employment: How Susceptible Are Jobs to Computerisation?', September 2013 www.oxfordmartin.ox.ac.uk/downloads/academic/The_Future_of_Employment.pdf

39 'The Side Hustle Economy', July 2018, assets.henley.ac.uk/defaultUploads/PDFs/news/Journalists-Regatta-Henley_Business_School_whitepaper_DIGITAL.pdf?mtime=20180703154430&_ga=2.120242955.240996529.1532257388-827778871.1532257388

40 Kollewe, Julia, 'Quarter of households in UK will rent privately by end of 2021, says report', *Guardian*, 12 June 2017

41 'Childbearing for women born in different years, England and Wales: 2016', 24 November 2017 www.ons.gov.uk/peoplepopulationandcommunity/birthsdeathsandmarriages/conceptionandfertilityrates/bulletins/childbearingforwomenbornindifferentyearsenglandandwales/2016

42 'Gig economy: time to shift the spotlight to older self-employed workers', 3 October 2017, www.ageing-better.org.uk/news/gig-economy-time-shift-spotlight-older-self-employed-workers

43 'An agile learning mindset is the only way you'll own your own future', 11 May 2017, www.seattletimes.com/opinion/an-agile-learning-mindset-is-the-only-way-youll-own-your-own-future/

44 '"I'm getting a big buzz out of it": five former professionals on their first term teaching', 11 Mar 2018, www.theguardian.com/education/2018/mar/11/im-getting-a-big-buzz-former-professionals-teaching-lucy-kellaway-now-teach

45 'The strange case of the death of friendship', 7 Nov 2001, www.independent.co.uk/arts-entertainment/books/news/the-strange-case-of-the-death-of-friendship-9137637

46 'Loneliness – What characteristics and circumstances are associated with feeling lonely?', 10 April 2018, www.ons.gov.uk/peoplepopulationandcommunity/wellbeing/articles/lonelinesswhatcharacteristicsandcircumstancesareassociatedwithfeelinglonely/2018-04-10

47 CIGNA US Loneliness Index: Survey of 20,000 Americans examining behaviors driving loneliness in the United States', May 2018, www.multivu.com/players/English/8294451-cigna-us-loneliness-survey/

48 'Facebook expects half of employees to work remotely over next five to 10 years', 21 May 2020, www.theguardian.com/technology/2020/may/21/facebook-coronavirus-remote-working-policy-extended-years

49 'Morgan Stanley CEO sees a future for the bank with "much less real estate"', 16 April 2020, www.bloomberg.com/news/articles/2020-04-16/gorman-sees-morgan-stanley-future-with-much-less-real-estate

50 'Working from home and coronavirus: Pyjama-clad remote workers are reluctant to return to the office', 16 April 2020, inews.co.uk/news/working-from-home-coronavirus-remote-workers-self-isolation-office-commute-419291

51 'Collaboration During Coronavirus: The Impact of COVID-19 on the Nature of Work', July 2020, www.nber.org/papers/w27612

52 'The Implications of Working Without an Office', 15 July 2020, hbr.org/2020/07/the-implications-of-working-without-an-office

53 'Gender Discrepancies in the Outcomes of Schedule Control on Overtime Hours and Income in Germany', 17 August 2016, academic.oup.com/esr/article/32/6/752/2525493?s=03

54 'Conspicuous Consumption of Time: When Busyness and Lack of Leisure Time Become a Status Symbol', 27 December 2016, academic.oup.com/jcr/article/44/1/118/2736404

55 'The reason Zoom calls drain your energy', 22 April 2020, www.bbc.com/worklife/article/20200421-why-zoom-video-chats-are-so-exhausting

56 'Remote Work Can Bring Benefits, but Attitudes Are Divided', 14 November 2018, www.indeed.com/lead/remote-work-survey

57 'Working mothers interrupted more often than fathers in lockdown – study', 27 May 2020, The Institute for Fiscal Studies and the UCL Institute of Education www.theguardian.com/world/2020/may/27/working-mothers-interrupted-more-often-than-fathers-in-lockdown-study

58 'UK working mothers are "sacrificial lambs" in coronavirus childcare crisis', 24 July 2020, www.theguardian.com/money/2020/jul/24/uk-working-mothers-are-sacrifical-lambs-in-coronavirus-childcare-crisis

59 'Women's research plummets during lockdown - but articles from men increase', 12 May 2020, www.theguardian.com/education/2020/may/12/womens-research-plummets-during-lockdown-but-articles-from-men-increase

60 'Why take-up of shared parental leave is so dismally low – and the solution', 20 November 2019, www.cityam.com/why-take-up-of-shared-parental-leave-is-so-dismally-low-and-how-to-fix-it/

61 'Working from..? A quick poll on virtual and office-based working', 23 July 2020, www.linkedin.com/pulse/working-from-quick-poll-virtual-office-based-perry-timms/?published=t

62 'The TWaT revolution: office on Tuesday, Wednesday and Thursday only', 19 January 2020, www.spectator.co.uk/article/the-twat-revolution-office-on-tuesday-wednesday-and-thursday-only

63 'The Eggs of Price: An Ovo-Urban Analogy', 3 October 2011, bigthink.com/strange-maps/534-the-eggs-of-price-an-ovo-urban-analogy

64 'Why your "weak-tie" friendships may mean more than you think', 3 July 2020 www.bbc.com/worklife/article/20200701-why-your-weak-tie-friendships-may-mean-more-than-you-think

65 'How Pixar Fosters Collective Creativity', September 2008 hbr.org/2008/09/how-pixar-fosters-collective-creativity

66 'Thought Leadership 2016 – Evolution of the Workplace Part 1', 2016, paramountinteriors.com/blog/thought-leadership-2016-%E2%80%93-evolution-of-the-workplace-part-1

CHAPTER OPENER QUOTATIONS

Page 1 'Phenomenal Woman', Maya Angelou

Page 12 *Oh the Thinks You Can Think*, Dr Seuss

Page 44 '9 To 5', Dolly Parton

Page 82 Cher to Jane Pauley, *Dateline*, 1996

Page 114 Unattributed

Page 142 Unattributed

Page 174 'The pandemic is a portal', Arundhati Roy, *The Financial Times*, April 2020

Page 200 Alvin Toffler, *FutureShock*, 1970

ACKNOWLEDGEMENTS

Thank you to the dear friends and family who waded through early drafts: Andy, Robert, Pauline and Daniel Auerbach, Andrea Lyttleton, Katie Churcher, Marina Camiletti, Jenny and David Silverman, Adam Chmielowski, Annie Crombie, Tammy Reynolds and especially Ben Lyttleton.

Thanks to the friends and expert colleagues whose ears I bent (flexed) and who gave me such interesting perspectives: Anthony Bale, Zoe Bloom, Daisy Donovan, Helen Dwyer, Sarah Galgey, Annie Gallimore, Cindy Gallop, Emma Gannon, Pinny Grylls, Sarah Hesz, Katharine Hill, Jules McKeen, Timothy Philips, Miriam Rayman, Kate Shepherd Cohen, Anniki Sommerville, Dale Southerton, Jan Toledano, Amelia Torode, Mark Williamson, Avivah Wittenberg-Cox and Rosie and Faris Yakob.

And huge thanks to the amazingly talented team at HQ: Lisa Milton, Kate Fox, Joe Thomas, Liz Marvin, Jen Callahan Packer, Noleen Robinson, Jo Surman, Charlie Redmayne.

MUSEUM MYSTERY SQUAD

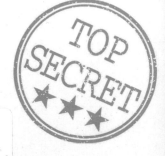

To Joseph and Theo, remembering our times
exploring the National Museum of Scotland – M.N.

To Hannah – M.P.

Kelpies is an imprint of Floris Books
First published in 2018 by Floris Books

The publisher acknowledges subsidy from
Creative Scotland towards the publication
of this volume

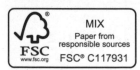

MIX
Paper from
responsible sources
FSC® C117931

 Also available as an eBook

British Library CIP data available
ISBN 978-178250-364-4
Printed & bound by MBM Print SCS Ltd, Glasgow

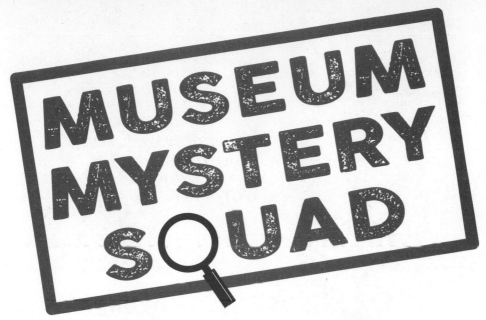

and the Case of the
Roman Riddle

Written by Mike Nicholson

Illustrated by Mike Phillips

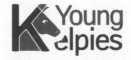

Young Kelpies

THE SQUAD

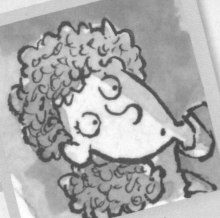

Kennedy

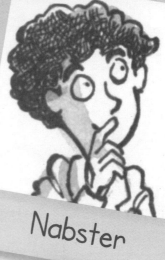

Nabster

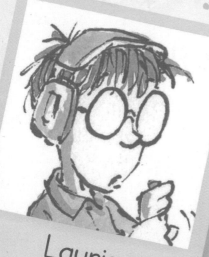

Laurie

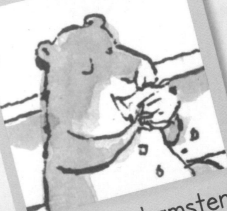

Colin the hamster

AND FEATURING...

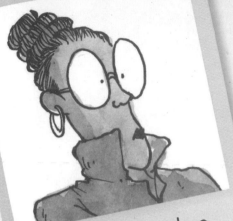

Saskia Spectre

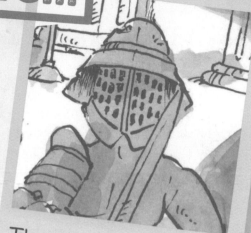

The Ghostly Gladiator

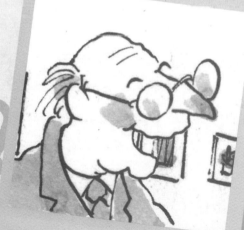

Joking Jimmy

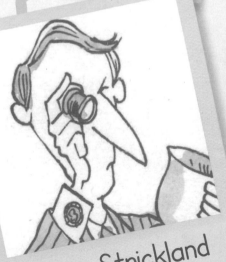

Angus Strickland

Some people think that museums are boring places.

Glass cases. Old stuff. Dust.

Wrong.

Think more of

wild animals

ANCIENT MUMMIES

enormous insects

COLOURFUL COSTUMES

glittering treasure

and amazing objects found nowhere else in the world.

Then imagine that each thing in the museum has its own strange story. With secrets from the past to be uncovered. Codes to be cracked. Odd characters and their fiendish plans. Each one creating a job for a team of expert investigators:

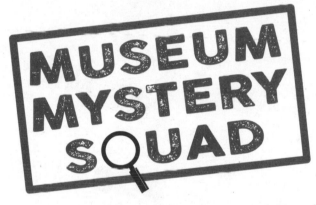

In this book you will find the Squad in the depths of the museum, somewhere in a maze of corridors and stairs.

Today, like every day, they have a puzzle to solve...

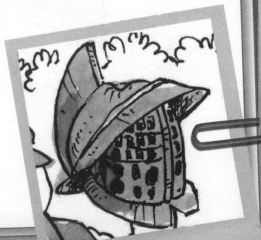

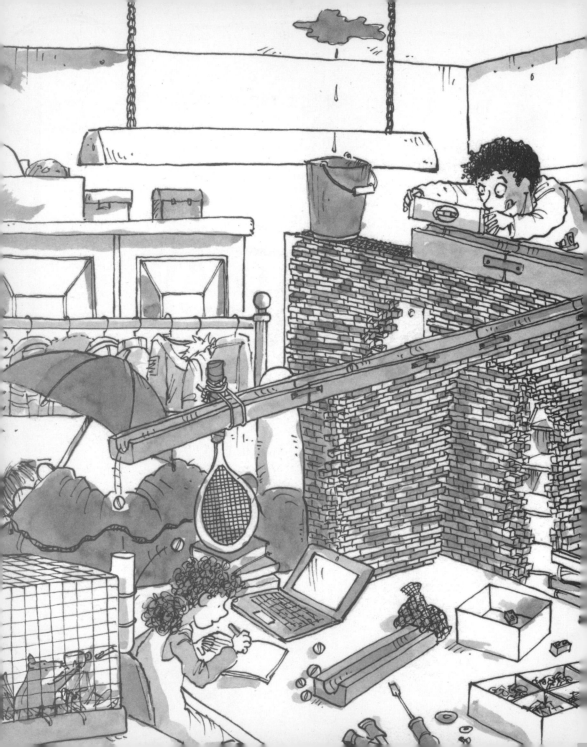

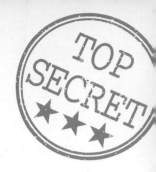

Chapter 1
In which things
unexpectedly get wet

"Ummm, Nabster, what exactly is this?" Kennedy Kerr

had been busy doodling in her diary. Looking up, she'd

discovered that the Museum Mystery Squad headquarters

was being taken over by a new construction. Balanced

above it on a ladder was the Squad's technical and

fix-it expert, Mohammed McNab (known to most people

as Nabster). Staring at the arches and bridges, Kennedy

went on, "Are you building an entire city in here?"

"It's just some Lego with the chutes from my

marble run," Nabster answered her, distracted by measuring the slope. "And I've also used that pile of books there. Oh, and that old tennis racquet. I was running out of Lego, you see, so I had to improvise."

"Right..." Kennedy clearly felt there was more to explain here. "Is it a very wide skyscraper?" she asked, checking they could still actually get to the HQ door.

"Noooo, think back about 2,200 years before the skyscraper was invented."

"Pyramid? No... temple? Roman Colosseum?"

"Decent guess! Yes, it's Roman, but not a Colosseum. When I heard that it will take a week for the museum janitor to fix the leaky pipe dripping through our ceiling, I decided we might as well use the water. And the Romans gave me an idea."

Kennedy's eyes lit up. "An aqueduct! Is that what it is?"

"Yep! I've just got to create a perfectly even slope along the top of it so the water keeps flowing. I'm testing it with marbles." Nabster put down his spirit level and ran two more marbles down the chute.

"Once it's finished, where will the water actually go?"

Nabster pointed to the cage in one corner of the room. Inside it Colin the hamster snuffled about in his straw, not realising the latest invention in the room was for him.

"I thought our leak could top up Colin's water feeder. Gets rid of one daily chore..." Nabster was pleased with his plan.

"As long as you keep any drips away from me," said a voice from the sofa. "There's nothing worse than a soggy sleeping bag." When there weren't mysteries to solve,

Laurie Lennox believed in catching up on a bit of sleep. Yet somehow he tuned in to any vital discussions in the HQ.

"I promise no drips, Laurie," said Nabster. "Aqueducts were one of the Romans' finest inventions!"

"Did *they* make them out of marble runs and sports equipment too?" asked Laurie.

"Aqueducts *are* a very clever idea," remarked Kennedy. "It's like having a river flow over a bridge instead of under it. You can use them to send water wherever you want."

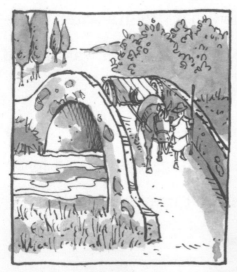

bridge

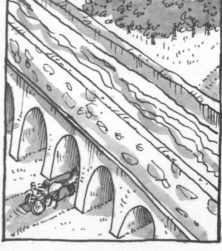

aqueduct

"Exactly," said Nabster. "The Romans moved water miles from the mountains, through hills, across valleys, to the city – keeping the same gentle slope on the aqueduct all the way. I'm going to take these drips from the ceiling to Colin's cage, but I'm testing it first with marbles. Once I put the bottom piece of chute in, Colin can have running water."

This was classic Nabster. If he didn't have a gadget to play with, he would just create his own inventions out of whatever was lying around.

Kennedy watched as he connected a piece of chute at the top, right under the constant drip in the ceiling.

Laurie's head stretched out of his sleeping bag, like a meerkat peering out of a hole in the ground. He began rummaging through his wardrobe rail beside the sofa. "Remind me what the Romans wore?"

If Nabster could combine the strangest objects to make a gadget, Laurie could combine the oddest clothes to make an outfit. He could mix and match stripy wellies, a tuxedo and a tiger-print shirt and somehow make it look good.

Nabster looked down from his ladder. "If you want to dress Roman style you could always just wrap yourself in a sheet and call it a toga."

"That'd be perfect for you, Laurie!" remarked Kennedy. "You could walk around in bedclothes all day."

"Ha ha." Laurie picked out some leather sandals. "These might be good if we get any puddles in here." He pointed to the table, where a small pool of water was starting to form beside Nabster's laptop.

"NO!" Nabster dived to save his things from the mini waterfall.

"Water dripping on a laptop?" Kennedy laughed. "That's one problem the Romans never had to deal with!"

As Nabster gently wiped his computer dry and carried it to a safer place, it made a familiar noise:

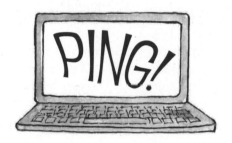

"There's a coincidence," he said, checking the new message in the Squad's inbox. It was an email from Magda Gaskar, the Museum Director, asking the Museum Mystery Squad to take on a new investigation, and this one was in the Roman Zone.

Dear Kennedy, Laurence and Mohammed,

Something strange is going on. I'd like you to look into it.

Three different visitors to the Roman Zone have told staff that they got a fright when the gladiator figure in our display spoke to them. Very odd! And yesterday a tour group were so spooked that the whole busload left the museum screaming about a ghost. Apparently they saw strange green smoke coming from the same figure.

Frankly, the idea that there is anything ghostly in the Roman Zone is ridiculous, but unless we can find out what's really going on, I will get rid of the gladiator. It's only a trial display, and I want crowds in the museum for the right reasons – not because we're making headlines for being haunted!

16

"Haunted?" scoffed Nabster. "What rubbish! I don't believe in ghosts. There has to be another explanation."

He rapidly finished off the aqueduct, moving the last piece of chute into place above Colin's water feeder, then he got out his equipment bag. He looked at the items he usually packed for an investigation: electronic measuring tape, string, bits of wire, pliers... Would any of these help prove that this gladiator ghost *wasn't* a ghost?

17

He decided to pack:

· the ScanRay (no matter what Magda was asking, Nabster's favourite gadget went everywhere)

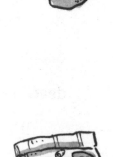

· his notebook

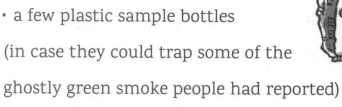

· a pencil

· the camera

· some popcorn (because solving mysteries makes you hungry)

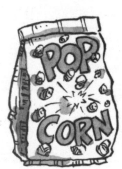

· a few plastic sample bottles (in case they could trap some of the ghostly green smoke people had reported)

· and the bag of marbles (because they'd helped in testing the aqueduct's slope and an inventor never knows when even the strangest things might come in useful again).

18

While Nabster gathered things up, Laurie was thinking. "You say the idea it's a ghost is rubbish? I'm not so sure. Every ancient object has been handled by people over the centuries, and all those people are now dead. That's kind of spooky!"

"It's true," nodded Kennedy. "The museum contains thousands of old things, and all of them have their stories from the past."

"Yeah, there are dead people's fingerprints on everything upstairs!" Laurie's eyes widened behind his glasses.

"That doesn't make them haunted," said Nabster, dismissing the idea. "No matter how old or strange an object is, there's no such thing as ghosts." He clipped the top of his bag firmly shut. "We'll do a proper investigation and find out what's really happening."

"Sounds good to me. Let's go!" Kennedy shut her diary and dashed beneath an aqueduct arch, leaving the door to the HQ swinging open and the sound of running footsteps disappearing down the corridor. Whenever there was a new mystery to solve, Kennedy was super-quick: she thought fast, and had extra-speedy feet too.

Nabster grabbed his equipment bag and followed swiftly. Last out the door was Laurie. He'd stopped to drape a sheet around himself like a toga, only to find that sprinting and wearing a robe do not go well together.

Colin watched each of them leave and took a sip from the trickle of water that had finally completed the long journey down the aqueduct to his feeder. He had always

managed to be an unexpectedly useful member of the
Museum Mystery Squad when they'd solved cases in the
past, but aqueducts, togas, gladiators and ghosts didn't
mean much to him. As he lay down in his straw for a
nap, it wasn't clear how he could possibly help this time.

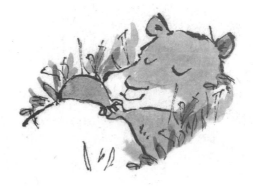

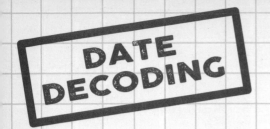

The Romans used a system of letters to write down numbers. Can you help Kennedy figure out these important dates from history using these Roman numerals?

KEY

I	=	1	IX	=	9	LXXX	=	80
II	=	2	X	=	10	XC	=	90
III	=	3	XII	=	12	C	=	100
IV	=	4	XX	=	20	D	=	500
V	=	5	XXX	=	30	DCCC	=	800
VI	=	6	XL	=	40	CM	=	900
VII	=	7	L	=	50	M	=	1000
VIII	=	8	LX	=	60	MM	=	2000

EXAMPLE:

MCML =   M   +   CM   +   L

1000 +   900   +   50   = 1950

First Roman invasion of Britain

$L + V$

___ + ___ = [ ] B.C.

Battle of Hastings

$M + LX + VI$

_____ + _____ + _____ = [ ]

Mary Queen of Scots is executed

$M + D + LXXX + VII$

_____ + _____ + _____ + _____ = [ ]

Queen Victoria becomes queen

$M + DCCC + XXX + VII$

_____ + _____ + _____ + _____ = [ ]

End of the First World War

$M + CM + X + VIII$

_____ + _____ + _____ + _____ = [ ]

Astronaut Neil Armstrong walks on the Moon

$M + CM + LX + IX$

_____ + _____ + _____ + _____ = [ ]

One of the three Olympics held in London

$MM + XII$

_____ + _____ = [ ]

ANSWERS ON THE LAST PAGE

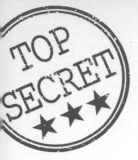
Chapter 2
In which 24 hours
sounds like a very long time

By the time Laurie and Nabster had run through the

many corridors under the museum and climbed the

maze of stairs to the main exhibition area, Kennedy

had already entered the Roman Zone. Inside, the

floor was covered in marble tiles. Columns and arches

divided the space, which was packed with pots and

plates, coins and clothes, and warriors with weapons.

Laurie's eye was immediately drawn to life-size

figures of Roman soldiers, all wearing sandals matching his,

24

along with bright red tunics and shiny body armour.

"I'd like one of those," he said, pointing to the impressive crested headgear worn by a centurion.

Nabster scanned it and, weirdly, the ScanRay told him the fancy brush on top was made from:

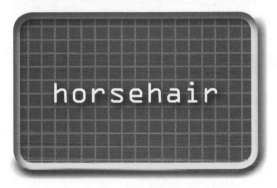

horsehair

He moved on to a giant table map of Britain behind the centurion, and pressed buttons to turn on lines of tiny lights. These showed where massive walls built by the Romans stretched right across parts of England and Scotland, from the east coast to the west.

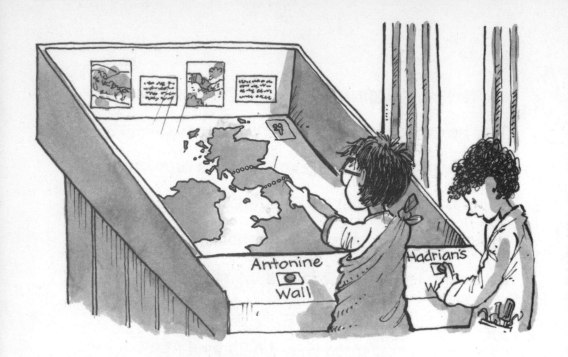

"Wow! 73 miles long and a castle every mile?" Laurie was looking over his friend's shoulder. "You were right Nabster, the Romans were amazing at building things, although I haven't seen an aqueduct for a hamster yet."

"It's just as well Colin's not with us. What would he think of that?" commented Nabster, pointing to a huge and ferocious stuffed leaping tiger. Standing ready to fight the attacking beast was a gladiator, one of Rome's specially trained fighters.

Kennedy approached it. "So this must be the ghostly gladiator." A metal helmet with a grid-like visor completely hid its face, making the figure seem strangely sinister.

The gladiator stood poised to defend itself: sword arm raised, the other hand clutching a heavy net that drooped down to the floor beside its leather sandals. It appeared all set for a fight to the death.

"Woah," said Kennedy, reading the information board next to the display. "It says here gladiators could be thrown into the arena with tigers, lions, bears or even crocodiles!"

Nabster climbed on a footstool to get a closer look. He leaned round to peer through the gladiator's visor. "BOO!" he said. There was no response. "Well, there's not a hint of smoke and I certainly can't hear any odd voices." He had found exactly what he had expected: nothing.

The Squad's inspection of the gladiator was interrupted by Gus, their good friend and the museum's security guard.

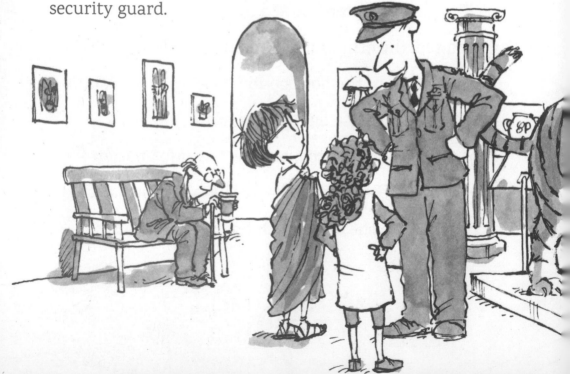

"I thought you lot might be here," he said. "Very strange one this. Very strange indeed." His eyes widened and he put on a spooky voice. **"CAN YOU FE-E-EEL THE GHO-O-OSTLY PRESENCE!?"**

Laurie held his breath. With Gus there was always a risk – a big risk. Was he going to tell one of his famously bad jokes? Of *course* he was.

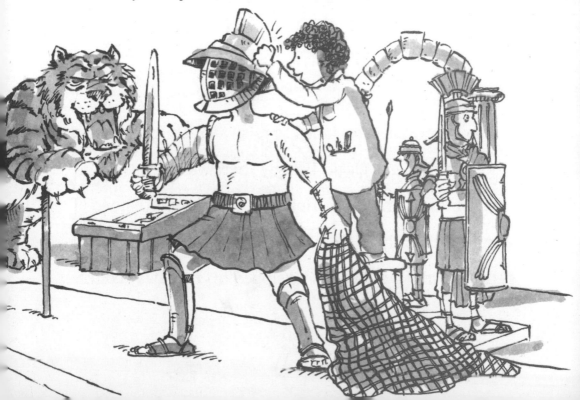

"That's what phantoms give each other at Christmas!"
Gus grinned and nudged Laurie so hard he nearly fell
over. "Get it? Presence... presents... ghostly *presence*?"

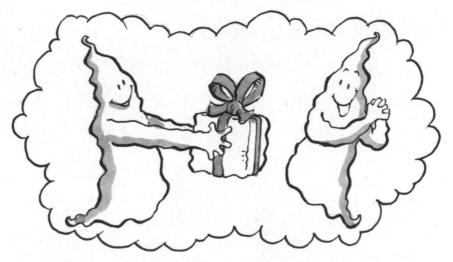

Usually Gus's jokes failed to raise a laugh from anyone
– not even a slight giggle. Usually there was silence, or
sometimes a faint groan. However, this time it seemed
someone actually found his joke amusing. An elderly man
sitting nearby guffawed as he sipped his takeaway coffee.

"That's a good one that is," he called over with a grin. "Ghostly presence!" Gus looked pleased to have found an audience who appreciated him, even if it was a very small one.

Exact size of joke-appreciating audience	Exact size of joke-UN-appreciating audience
1	3

The man raised his coffee as if to say 'Cheers!'

"Oh no," whispered Laurie. "Gus is getting some encouragement!"

Sure enough, Gus decided to have another go. "What do you call a big building with lots of scary displays and exhibits inside?"

He looked at the Squad, who all shrugged. "A BOO-seum! Get it? Like a *mu*-seum but scary... BOO!"

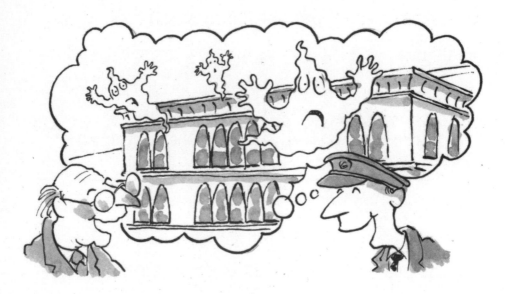

Nabster closed his eyes tight, as if wishing the moment would end.

It didn't, because the old man with the coffee laughed again. "Ha! Boo-seum!" he chuckled as he repeated Gus's joke.

"I have to admit," said Gus. "That was a frightful joke! Get it...? *Fright*–full... full of fright?"

The man chuckled and raised his cup again.

Kennedy bravely stepped in to save them all from the unfolding nightmare of more Gus jokes.

"So, talking of frights, Gus, do you know what's been happening here?"

Her question turned Gus from bad comedian to professional security guard in an instant. He straightened his cap and began to explain. Apparently the spooky events had taken place at random times of day, and, as Magda's email had said, involved eerie green smoke coming from the gladiator's helmet as well as a voice in a strange language that no one understood.

"Fascinating!" said Laurie. "Out of all the ancient bones, creatures and clothes in this building, something *must* be haunted. So maybe we have a two-thousand-year-old gladiator who's decided to come back and reclaim his old armour or helmet!"

"Even if things are old or dead, it doesn't make them haunted," said Nabster firmly. "Most stories of haunted places are just inspired by creaking floors and squeaky doors. Some people have overactive imaginations! I don't believe in any ghostly gladiator. It's time for some proper answers." He switched on the ScanRay and was about to point it at the gladiator's helmet when Magda Gaskar, the Museum Director, marched into the room like she meant business.

"Ah good, I'm glad to see you're all here. Things are

moving very quickly. I've just
been told that the cleaners
are refusing to come in at
the usual time tomorrow
before the museum opens."

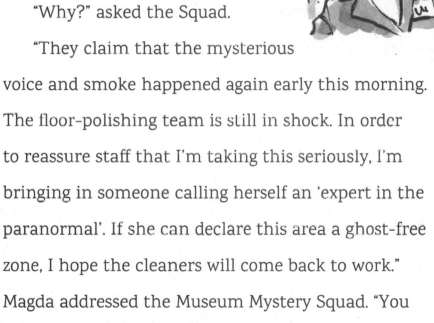

"Why?" asked the Squad.

"They claim that the mysterious
voice and smoke happened again early this morning.
The floor-polishing team is still in shock. In order
to reassure staff that I'm taking this seriously, I'm
bringing in someone calling herself an 'expert in the
paranormal'. If she can declare this area a ghost-free
zone, I hope the cleaners will come back to work."
Magda addressed the Museum Mystery Squad. "You
three should carry on with your investigation as well.

The more people trying to solve this, the better."

"Expert in the paranormal?" Laurie's eyes lit up. "A ghost hunter! How exciting!"

"Not when she doesn't find anything," murmured Nabster.

"Never mind about her," said Kennedy. "Let's concentrate on our own work. Gus says that these strange events are happening at random times – which means we can't predict when the gladiator will speak or smoke next..."

"I smell bad news coming," Nabster groaned.

"...So, to make sure we're in the Roman Zone for the ghost's next appearance, I propose a 24-hour watch," finished Kennedy.

"Night of the Ghost Watch! Brilliant! Even I can stay

awake for that!" grinned Laurie.

Nabster wasn't so enthusiastic. "A whole night without sleep... waiting for something that doesn't exist!"

Gus grinned. "Sounds fun. I bet you'll have a wail of a time! Get it? 'Whale of a time' but with ghosts... wail... Wail of a time?"

Smiling weakly at Gus's latest effort, the Squad left him and his elderly audience of one chuckling together, as they headed back to the aqueduct-filled HQ to plan their spooky stakeout.

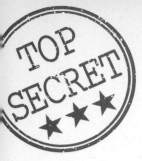

Chapter 3
In which a ploughed field produces a surprise

Sitting under the gently flowing aqueduct, Kennedy, Nabster and Laurie discussed the case. Something strange was definitely going on in the Roman Zone, and hopefully on their overnight watch they'd be the next people to hear and see it.

Laurie kept coming back to the idea that the figure really was haunted. "Everyone who's heard the voice thinks there's a ghost. What if there really is?" He was, as usual, in his sleeping bag on the sofa, but he was very much awake.

Nabster was impatient. "Ghosts *don't* exist. There *has* to be an explanation."

"We should at least consider it, Nabster," said Kennedy. "We wouldn't be doing our job properly if we didn't."

"OK then, so in stories about ghosts, why do places get haunted?" asked Laurie. "What is it that causes dead people to come back as ghosts?"

Kennedy stepped through an aqueduct arch to start a giant mind map on the smartboard. Laurie and Nabster moved to watch. Ideas were soon coming thick and fast.

"Well, ghosts are scary, so maybe they just enjoy frightening people?" Kennedy suggested.

Laurie frowned. "Or they could be warning people off? Sometimes you hear stories about ghosts keeping people away from something... or somewhere."

39

"What if a ghost was out for revenge?" Nabster offered reluctantly.

"That's a good one." Kennedy added it to the board. "Most gladiators died in fights with other gladiators or with wild animals. Maybe ours isn't too happy about that?"

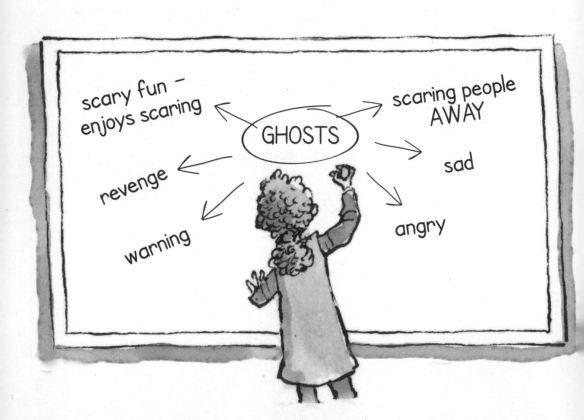

"Some gladiators were far from home." Laurie remembered what they'd read on the information boards upstairs. "They'd been captured and become slaves and made to fight. There are lots of reasons for them to be unhappy or want to make someone sorry."

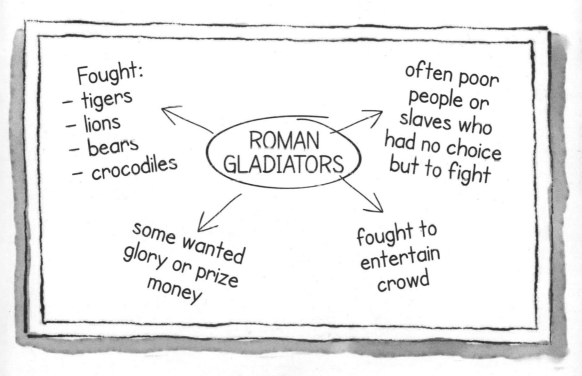

Fought:
- tigers
- lions
- bears
- crocodiles

ROMAN GLADIATORS

often poor people or slaves who had no choice but to fight

some wanted glory or prize money

fought to entertain crowd

"Nice idea," said Nabster, "But our *supposed* gladiator ghost upstairs is mumbling nonsense and spewing out weird green smoke. How is that getting revenge? And on who?"

"Well if it wants to scare people away then it's doing a good job." Kennedy sat back down. "According to Magda, the cleaners are already steering clear. If word gets out then the museum might have fewer visitors – who wants a nice family day out that ends with everyone being scared stiff?"

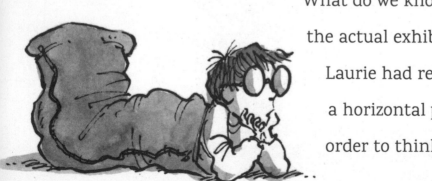

"What do we know about the actual exhibit then?" Laurie had returned to a horizontal position in order to think better.

"Well it looked pretty normal to me," said Nabster. "I never got round to scanning any of it, but there were no signs of smoke or noise."

"But what do we *actually* know about it?" asked Laurie. "Like how old is the gladiator armour? Magda said the figure is a trial display. Where did it come from?" Laurie was known for asking direct questions, and this habit showed no sign of disappearing.

Nabster began searching on the laptop. Kennedy moved to look over his shoulder. Within a couple of minutes he had discovered that the gladiator helmet and some of the other Roman items upstairs had only arrived in the museum two weeks ago.

"The Taggart Treasure," read Kennedy.

"What's that?" The word 'treasure' caused Laurie to sit up again eagerly. He was imagining swinging a big sword covered in jewels.

"Some of the objects in the Roman Zone were found by a farmer in a field just last year," Kennedy explained.

"Mr James Taggart of Taggart Farm, West Lothian, to be precise," Nabster read aloud from his laptop screen. "He ploughed them up!"

"What were the Romans doing in West Lothian?" asked Laurie.

"Well, they built one of those long walls there," said Nabster. "Remember, it was on that table map with the buttons and lights upstairs: the Antonine Wall."

Nabster clicked on a news item about the Roman discovery on the farm. The screen filled with the face of a woman being interviewed. The chatty farmer had clearly spent lots of time outdoors; her face was nut brown, with shiny red cheeks. The caption underneath identified her as 'Rosie Taggart'.

"Well, there was quite a clunk when it happened," she explained. The camera pulled back to show the woman holding a metal helmet.

"That's the gladiator helmet upstairs!" shouted Nabster.

45

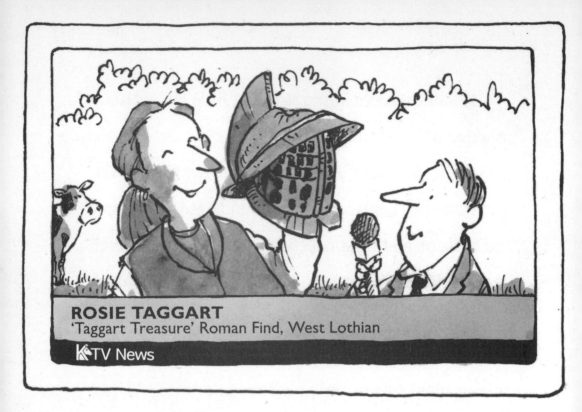

ROSIE TAGGART
'Taggart Treasure' Roman Find, West Lothian

TV News

The interview continued. "My dad, James Taggart, was ploughing this field and heard a thud. He looked back and saw a metal lump lying behind the tractor, and when he jumped out to check, he found this helmet. I think the dent in the top was probably from the impact of the plough!"

The film showed vast fields bordered by hedges, and a town in the distance, as well as farm sheds with straw-covered floors. The farm had only ever been famous for its tatties and an annual Fireworks Festival that took place in the field, said Rosie Taggart, but the discovery of the helmet had changed all that. There had been huge interest, and a massive dig had been organised with dozens of volunteers, which led to more ancient items being uncovered: jewellery, coins and some weapons too. "The whole lot is now called the 'Taggart Treasure'," finished Rosie proudly.

As the film clip ended, Laurie asked, "So did the farmer give it all to the museum?"

Kennedy scanned the screen for more information. "Not exactly. It's treasure trove."

47

"Treasure trove? Isn't that to do with pirates?" joked Nabster.

"It's what important historical items like these are called if they're found unexpectedly. By law they get described as 'treasure' and the museum has a chance to buy them so that everyone can see them."

"You mean if you find treasure you don't get to keep it?" Laurie's visions of himself dressed in gold and jewels suddenly vanished.

"Well, if you don't, you're given money for it," explained Kennedy. "This museum is still deciding whether to buy the Taggart Treasure. It's been valued and put on display." She was now reading from the museum website. "Magda wanted to see whether people were interested in it."

48

"She wasn't expecting they might be scared off by it!" said Laurie.

"No," said Kennedy. "If it keeps happening, I guess the Taggart Treasure won't be bought for the museum's permanent collection."

An image of the gladiator's helmet now filled the wall screen. The dent in the top was clear to see.

"What if the gladiator is unhappy because his helmet has been bashed?" wondered Lauric. "An angry ghost, annoyed with people for damaging his armour!"

Nabster sighed. "You just don't give up do you?"

"We can argue about this later," interrupted Kennedy. "Right now we need to get organised for our 24-hour watch. So far, any appearance has involved a voice and smoke. Nabster, can you bring some kit to

49

record sounds and capture anything in the air?"

"I've got empty bottles already and I'll throw in a voice recorder in case Mr Ghost comes over all chatty. Happy?"

"Delighted!" Laurie jumped up and began to sift through his clothes rail for a ghost-hunting outfit. After thinking it over, he decided this was definitely a jumpsuit occasion. "Let's look at the other items in the

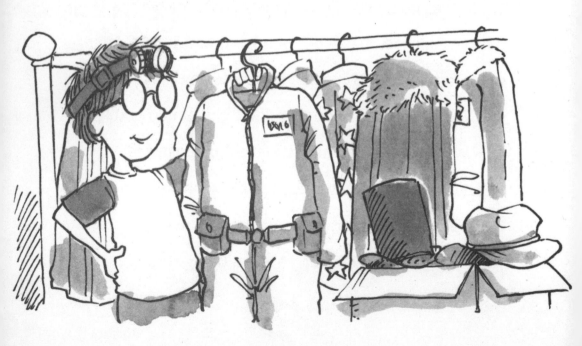

Taggart Treasure to check if they got bashed about on the farm too. It would be good to know just how angry this ghost might get!"

Nabster looked at his watch. "It's nearly closing time. We're going to be starting this watch as it gets dark."

"The perfect time to find a ghost!" said Kennedy.

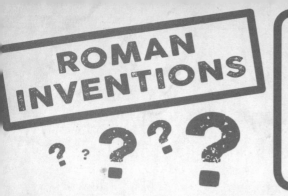

ROMAN INVENTIONS

? ? ?? ? ?

Nabster can't believe how many Roman inventions are still used today. Can you guess the answers to these Roman invention questions? Solutions at the back of the book!

Straight roads

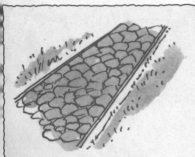

The Romans built long straight roads all over their empire. They were so well made, many still exist today, including in Britain, 2000 years later.

Why did the Romans want their roads to be straight?

Newspapers

Roman citizens could read about military victories, the times for gladiator fights, and important births and deaths in the *Acta Diurna* or 'daily acts' – an early kind of newspaper.

What were Roman newspapers made of?

Toilets

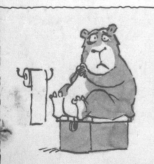

Ancient Rome was a very big city, and it had a sewage problem. Smelly! So the Romans invented flushing toilets and sewer pipes, to take the smelly stuff away from the city.

How did the Romans bring water into the city to flush all the toilets?

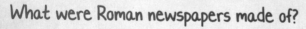

The Calendar

The Romans needed to number the days in a year, so they could make plans and coordinate across their big empire. The months we use today are based on their calendar, called the 'Julian' calendar. It was named after a famous Roman emperor.

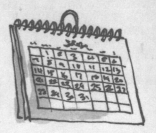

Can you guess the name of the famous Roman emperor?

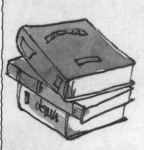

Books

Romans were the first civilisation to bind together pieces of paper to create a book. They called it a *caudex* (in English we say 'codex'), which also means 'tree trunk'.

Why did Romans use the same word for books and tree trunks?

The ScanRay

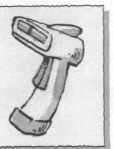

Hmmm, wait!

Did the Romans invent the ScanRay?

ANSWERS ON THE LAST PAGE

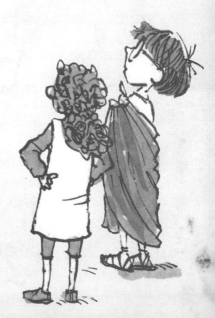

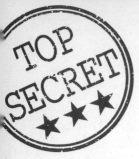
Chapter 4
In which Nabster is not snoring

Back upstairs in the Roman Zone, the Museum Mystery

Squad examined the other pieces of the Taggart

Treasure. There were coins with strange markings,

solid gold necklaces and silver drinking goblets. The

information board said it was very unusual to find a

gladiator's outfit so far from Rome. The objects from

the farmers' field were thought to have belonged

to a Roman general travelling in the British Isles.

Interesting, but the Squad couldn't see anything to

explain the recent ghostly activity.

They lay their sleeping bags beside some Roman columns, and settled down for 'Night of the Ghost Watch', as Laurie kept calling it. As the last light faded, the atmosphere in the Zone changed. The soldiers turned into shadowy silhouettes, and even the marble columns and arches took on a sinister appearance, looming above them in the darkness. Nothing moved, but everything somehow seemed as though it might. The team had been chatty before, but now they found themselves speaking in hushed tones.

"Everything looks so creepy," murmured Laurie, nervously glancing at the tiger. "I'm sure its eyes are following me. If one of its paws moves, I swear I'm out of here fast!"

"Laurie Lennox moving at speed? That'd be a first!"

Kennedy managed to joke, even though she felt a little uneasy too.

"This is exactly what I was talking about," Nabster shook his head. "At times like this your mind plays tricks on you. That's why people come up with ghost stories."

"But so far this ghost has only appeared to people in broad daylight, not the middle of the night," Kennedy reasoned. "Why would their minds be playing tricks on them in the day?"

Nabster had no answer for that. Instead, he yawned and curled up in a ball, clutching his equipment bag close like a big teddy bear. "Wake me up if it gets interesting."

"That's usually my line," whispered Laurie, shuffling

over to lean against a display case of Roman jewellery in the middle of the room, away from any dark corners. Kennedy joined him. It felt safer to sit together.

It was strange to be in the museum when it was so quiet. It was usually such a busy building. There were no echoing sounds of footsteps on the tiled floor. No doors opening. No chattering school children. Just... silence.

Kennedy and Laurie sat completely still, hardly daring to move. Eventually, Laurie had had enough and switched on his head torch, shining its spotlight slowly round the room. The beam reflected off the glass containers with their chipped plates and vases, and lit up the metal armour of the Roman soldiers. Nothing moved, and he turned it off again.

The darkness was still and silent, until...

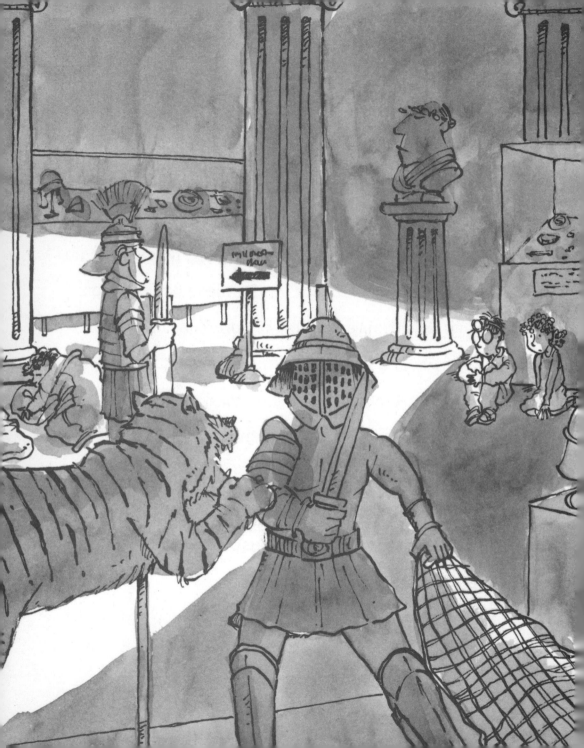

"What was that?" whispered Kennedy sharply.

"What?"

"Listen."

They strained to hear. Sure enough, there came a steady, rhythmical sound. The sound of... breathing.

In, out, in, out.

Their eyes widened. Who or *what* was in the room?

Laurie couldn't help but imagine an army of Roman warrior ghosts surrounding them in the darkness, swords raised.

Kennedy shook her head in annoyance. "It's just Nabster. Snoring in his sleep."

Laurie smiled in relief.

And then a voice spoke from the shadows.

Nabster's voice.

"I'm not snoring."

"What?"

"It's *not me*," Nabster repeated. "I'm as awake as you are!"

"Then... whose breathing is that?"

Laurie and Nabster froze, but Kennedy stood up cautiously. She listened hard, head to one side. "SSSHHH! Someone's speaking."

Hicnoloesse.

"Who said that?"

"Not me."

"Someone said something!"

Hicnoloesse.

Louder this time. Kennedy wasn't the only one on

60

her feet now. Nabster and Laurie stood on either side of her. Wide-eyed, all three Squad members listened again for another sound.

Hicnoloesse!

"Where is it coming from?" Laurie switched the torch on again and pointed it straight at the noise.

"It's the *gladiator*!" Kennedy cried.

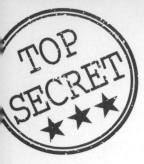

Chapter 5
In which it seems there are well-behaved snakes

"The gladiator can't be speaking!" said Nabster, though he didn't sound sure.

They all crept towards the figure of the fighter, inching forward.

Suddenly, there was a sharp **POP!** and a cloud of green smoke puffed from the holes in the gladiator's helmet.

Hicnoloesse! the voice boomed.

Still the smoke came, billowing around the

raised sword and through the mesh of the net in the gladiator's other hand. Laurie decided that the tiger wasn't so scary and stepped behind it, as if hoping the stuffed animal might protect him.

"Did that gladiator move?" He peered round the tiger's shoulder at the Roman warrior. "Did I see it move?"

Kennedy stood her ground, watching intently, trying to make sense of this surely impossible situation.

Ever the gadget-man, Nabster dived into his bag. In his panic the ScanRay fell to the floor, bits flying off in all directions. Ignoring the pain of seeing his precious invention in pieces, he quickly grabbed the voice recorder instead and turned it on.

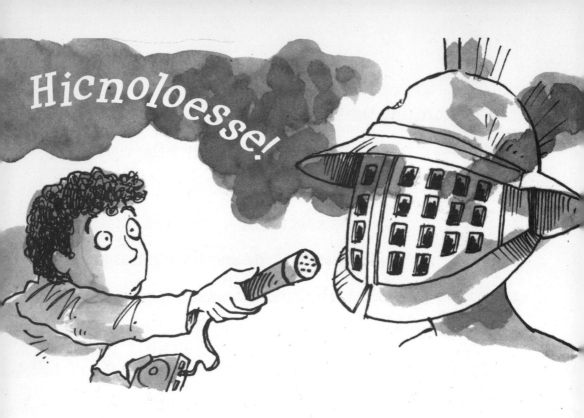

Hicnoloesse!

Hicnoloesse! repeated the voice as the eerie
green smoke began to disappear. Then just as Nabster
reached a perfect recording position in front of the
figure, it was all over. The smoke had dispersed. The
noise had stopped. The gladiator was just another
museum display once again.

"What just happened?!" asked Nabster in disbelief.

"That was intense... Totally freaky!" Laurie reappeared from behind the tiger.

"Have you ever seen anything like it?" asked Kennedy. Her eyes looked like they were out on stalks.

The others shook their heads in awe.

"If I was the cleaner here, I'd refuse to come back too," said Laurie. "That is one angry ghost!"

Kennedy looked up at the dark holes of the gladiator's helmet. "What was it saying?"

"It just sounded like nonsense to me," said Nabster. "Anyway, isn't the bigger question *how* was it speaking?"

All three Squad members were still in a slight state of shock when they heard the sound of approaching footsteps.

65

Whipping their heads round to check whether a centurion had gone for a late-night stroll, they were relieved to see Gus enter the room instead, dropping by to check on them with a flask of hot chocolate in hand.

"What's up with you lot?" he asked, looking at each Squad member in turn. "You all look like you've seen a ghost."

For once, Gus wasn't making a joke. It showed plainly on the team's faces that something very peculiar had happened. When Nabster filled him in on the spooky situation and played back the voice recording, Gus said he would report to Magda first thing in the morning.

"What will her 'expert in the paranormal' make of all this?" Kennedy wondered.

"She's due here at 11.00 a.m.," said Gus. "You should get some sleep and come back to the Roman Zone then."

"Good idea," nodded Laurie enthusiastically. Right now he could think of no better place than his safe, cosy sleeping bag – on a sofa that might be damp but definitely *wasn't* haunted.

Kennedy's Diary

Wednesday, midnight
Wow... What an end to the day, or is it the beginning of a new one? I've lost track!
OK, that was seriously WEIRD. Whether you believe in ghosts or not, the gladiator was really scary with all that swirling green smoke.

None of us have got a clue what his spooky voice said. It sounded something like 'hiccup lessons'. Or 'hockey lassies'? 'Tickle blessings'? It's a riddle - it makes no sense.

Nabster hasn't examined the voice recording yet. He's more concerned with trying to fix the ScanRay, which got broken in the chaos. At least the aqueduct is working well, thanks to all the testing with marbles. The drips are flowing smoothly now!

Laurie is so happy to be wrapped up in his sleeping bag, I'm not sure we'll ever see him again. Maybe meeting a real live ghost hunter will coax him back out!

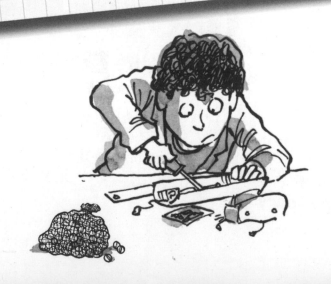

At 11.00 a.m. precisely, Magda Gaskar strode into the Roman

Zone, moments after the bleary-eyed Squad had arrived.

"I'd like you to meet Saskia Spectre," she announced.

"An expert with experience of... this type of situation."

If Laurie had big glasses, Saskia Spectre's were *so*

huge they looked like satellite dishes. Scrawled in red

on the back of her black bomber jacket were the words:

SASKIA SPECTRE
GHOST
HUNTER
MY NORMAL IS THE PARANORMAL

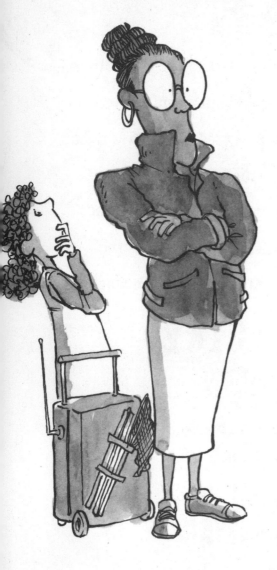

Topping off her look, Saskia's hair was twisted into a complicated plait, which was coiled high on her head like a nest of well-behaved snakes. Kennedy stared, wondering if her own wild hair could be tamed like that.

"Morning," Saskia greeted the group, sharply parking up a small suitcase on wheels in a business-like manner. "Until further notice, this is a **SUSPECTED SPOOK ZONE**. It's time to run some tests."

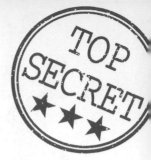

Chapter 6
In which there is a whiff of gadget

Nabster liked the idea of running tests. He stepped back and considered Saskia's suitcase. There was an aerial sticking out of one end, and attached to the side was a little fishing net with a folded, hinged pole. Like a dog catching the scent of a rabbit, Nabster was getting a distinct whiff of gadget. He hovered, hoping Saskia might open the suitcase to reveal ghoul-trapping goodies.

"Can you really catch ghosts with that fishing net?" asked Laurie curiously.

"You'd be surprised," replied Saskia.

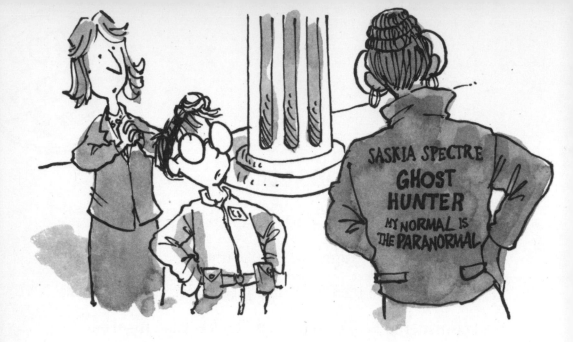

Laurie gave a look that suggested he would indeed.
He was slightly disappointed – he had expected a
real-life ghost hunter to wear a jumpsuit just like his.
Though he did rather like Saskia's bomber jacket.

Saskia started her enquiry. "Tell me exactly what
has been seen – or sensed – so far."

The Squad told the story of their night watch and
the ghost hunter nodded knowingly, slowly circling

the gladiator, pausing to peer into the tiger's jaws on the way past.

"It sounds like a classic stage 1 poltergeist. It's just warming up – letting you know it's here. If it progresses to stage 2, objects might start moving around." She gave them all a serious stare, her eyes like marbles in the lenses of her giant glasses. "In here, moving objects could be *very* dangerous." They all looked from the swords held by the Roman figures to the stuffed, leaping tiger, its face frozen in a ferocious snarl.

Laurie gulped.

"You said the ghost spoke," Saskia continued. "What *precisely* did it say?"

It was Kennedy who replied. "We couldn't make any sense of it. It was gobbledygook."

"That sounds like phantomese," said Saskia grimly.

"Is that even a language?" murmured Laurie.

Saskia began wafting her arms in a circular motion. "Right, next step is to connect with the atmosphere." Nabster stepped forwards hopefully, eager to see if she was going to plug something in. He was sorely disappointed when she simply took a deep breath and closed her eyes.

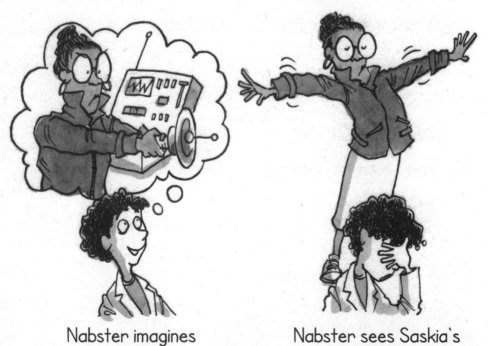

Nabster imagines
ghost hunting

Nabster sees Saskia's
actual ghost hunting

"I love those *spectre*-cles she's wearing!" whispered Gus. Laurie gave a slow, sad shake of his head, so Gus turned to look for appreciation elsewhere. There were no visitors allowed in the Roman Zone that morning, but a curious few had gathered by the barrier at the doorway, including the old man from the previous day, another coffee cup in hand. Gus put two circles of fingers up to his eyes like glasses and mouthed the word '*spectre*-cles' to him. The old man grinned and raised his cup to acknowledge the joke.

Eager to meet his one and only fan, Gus went over and they introduced themselves properly. The man was called Jimmy, and turned out to be visiting Edinburgh. He was staying nearby and enjoyed coming to the museum.

"I like sitting among all these amazing objects watching the world go by," said Jimmy, happily sipping his hot drink.

"Why don't you swap your coffee for some ghost food?" said Gus. "I hear they like I-*scream*! Get it? Ice cream... I-scream?"

"Never mind that," Jimmy grinned. "What game do ghosts like to play?... Hide and *shriek*!"

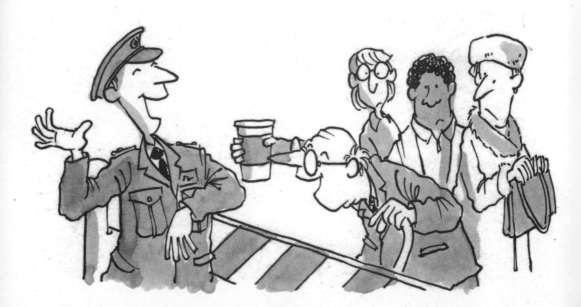

Soon Gus and Jimmy were swapping jokes and giggling like naughty schoolboys at the back of a classroom.

"Who won the skeleton beauty contest?... No-body!"

"Where do spooks buy stamps?... At the *ghost* office!"

"What kind of street do ghosts live on?... A dead end!"

Meanwhile, Saskia was still 'connecting with the atmosphere', breathing deeply and making a low hum. "Spirits can be stirred up by vibrations," she explained.

"You mean humming?" asked Laurie.

"Not *any* hum," said Saskia briskly. "Only the right frequency and tone."

She was now so close to the gladiator she was almost sniffing it. "Wait." She held up a hand to silence the room. "Listen... I hear a response!"

Saskia pulled up the suitcase aerial to maximum height, grabbed the net and snapped it open with one flick. The ghost hunter was ready to make a catch.

She tiptoed softly, as if stalking a butterfly, still humming and with her head to one side.

"I hear it humming back," she breathed.

Laurie moved closer. "Really?"

Kennedy's eyes widened. It seemed the ghost was about to speak again.

"Er... excuse me..." It was Nabster. "If it's humming you can hear... um... I think that might actually be... me." He held up the ScanRay guiltily. His gadget was making its usual buzzing noise. "Sorry! But the good news is it's working again!"

Saskia shoved the aerial roughly back down into

the case. "You're disrupting a *very* sensitive process."

Magda stepped forward, giving Nabster a serious look. "I can't have you getting in each other's way. Please give Saskia space to work."

"I'll take some readings elsewhere in the room," sniffed Saskia, wheeling her case further off. "I need to make sure you only have a problem in one area."

"Oh dear," said Magda nervously. "I do hope you don't find anything else. It's bad enough having people scared by *one* exhibit."

"I'm not so sure," said Gus quietly. "I think we should have more ghosts in the museum. I haven't had this much fun in ages. If other ghosts hear about this, they'll be dying to come here!... Dying... Ghosts... Dying to come here... Get it?"

Jimmy nearly toppled over laughing at that one and grabbed at his walking stick to steady himself.

As he did so, a man pushed past the small crowd gathered at the barrier. Gus stiffened and reached out an arm, keeping the entrance to the Roman Zone secure, but Magda waved him through.

"It's OK, Gus," she called. "This is Angus Strickland, everybody. He's responsible for deciding on the value of treasure discovered in Scotland. He spent some time assessing the Taggart Treasure after it was found. I invited him here to see it on display."

"He's a treasure trove guy!" Nabster looked impressed. "The person who works out how much money people are paid if the museum buys the stuff they find."

Angus Strickland looked sleek and smart in a crisp

pinstripe suit. His cufflinks were made of ancient-looking coins. The Squad watched as he made his way around the room eyeing up each object, his head twitching like a curious heron.

"Do you think each time he nods like that it means he's decided a price?" Laurie asked the others.

Strickland stopped as his eyes locked on the gladiator. "Here we are. Centrepiece of the Taggart Treasure. Good to see it in situ."

"Bless you," said Nabster.

"No, silly!" Kennedy smiled. "He didn't sneeze! He said 'in situ'. It's Latin – the language of ancient Rome."

Nabster looked confused. "What does 'in situ' mean?"

"'In the right place'," Kennedy explained. "The helmet is back on a gladiator instead of being in a muddy field."

Nabster shrugged. "Isn't it a bit odd to talk in a dead language?"

"Well, loads of English words we use all the time come from Latin," Kennedy told him. "Like 'ignorant' and 'language'."

Laurie was more interested in the gladiator's helmet. "So you've seen this treasure before?" he asked Strickland.

"Indeed," Strickland replied. "It's my job to check whether found objects are genuine, and to decide what they're worth."

"Is this worth a lot?" Laurie gestured to the helmet.

"Mmm." Strickland looked awkward, as if he didn't want to give away exact numbers. "Well, there are many factors to consider: the age, how rare the object is, if it's in good condition."

"This has a big bash from the plough," said Nabster.

"Yes, the damage by the farmer was unfortunate, but it means the museum will pay less, and that's good because it leaves more money to buy other treasure." He fingered the ancient coins on his cufflinks as he spoke. "I often think the small items are the real gems."

Magda interrupted to call Strickland to a museum meeting, and Gus went on with his rounds. Saskia continued wandering through the room 'connecting with the atmosphere'. The Squad found a quiet spot beside a centurion figure to discuss the progress of their investigation.

"OK, there's something I want to think about." Kennedy's brow was furrowed with concentration. "Laurie says there's a ghost, Nabster says not. Meanwhile, Magda really wants to prove there *isn't* one... What if there's someone who wants the opposite of that? Someone who really wants people to believe there *is* a ghost here?" She surveyed the room. Saskia was now humming loudly into a Roman urn. "Who *needs* ghosts?" Kennedy continued.

Laurie began to see what she was thinking. "A ghost hunter?"

"Exactly," Kennedy smiled. "When a ghost appears, ghost hunters get called in to sort them out."

"And they get paid to do it," said Nabster.

"So..." Laurie thought it through further. "If a ghost hunter *created* a ghost, she could make a nice little job for herself?"

"Correct again," said Kennedy.

"She could just bring in any old stuff and call it ghost-hunting equipment." Nabster frowned at the souped-up suitcase again. "And invent words like *phantomese.*"

"Are you saying she could then stop the pretend haunting and tell everyone she's got rid of the ghost?" asked Laurie.

"Exactly!" said Kennedy. "All eyes on Saskia Spectre. We watch her *every* move."

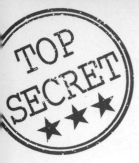

Chapter 7
In which both a suitcase
and a bottle are opened

Determined to keep eyes on Saskia at all times, the
Squad spent a good ten minutes watching the ghost
hunter's unusual methods, which now involved waving
a funnel in the air. It was joined onto a long vacuum-
cleaner tube that looped round twice before going
inside her suitcase. It looked as if she was trying to
hoover up a passing ghost from the air.

"Her ghost-hunting equipment is getting worse by
the minute." Nabster shook his head in disgust.

"It's all part of the act," replied Kennedy. "But she's about to get a little surprise." Saskia was walking backwards, concentrating hard on holding the funnel up high. "With ghost hunting," Kennedy said, grinning, "you just never know what's going to happen next…"

"I think I do," said Nabster, as Saskia took one more step back and toppled over her own suitcase. There was a windmill of arms, legs, fishing nets, aerials, tubes and suitcase handles and Saskia went down in a heap. As she did so, the case's lid sprung open with a sharp **CLICK** and everything spilled out.

"Yes!" Nabster pumped his fist in excitement. "We get to see what's inside!"

On her hands and knees, an embarrassed Saskia hurried to scoop up the scattered contents of her case.

87

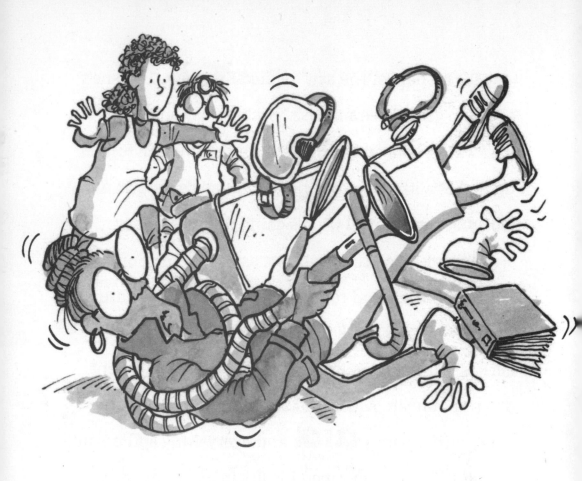

Kennedy rushed forward. "What a shame! Are you OK?

Let me help."

Realising this was a good way to get a closer look,

Laurie and Nabster quickly volunteered too. "Yeah, we'll give you a hand too!"

As they gathered the ghost hunter's belongings from the tiled floor, they realised the suitcase had contained quite an unusual collection of objects.

There were:

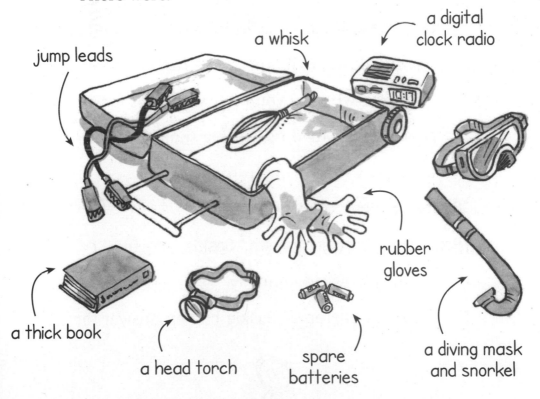

a digital clock radio

a whisk

jump leads

rubber gloves

a thick book

a head torch

spare batteries

a diving mask and snorkel

"So, this is what ghost-hunting equipment looks like," Kennedy commented chattily, pretending to brush dirt from Saskia's jacket.

Laurie was a little bit firmer in his questioning of their suspect: "These things are just any old bits and pieces, aren't they?"

Nabster, meanwhile, went in for the kill. "You can't possibly catch ghosts with any of this random stuff, can you? I mean, what do you use jump leads for?"

"To pass electric currents," Saskia snapped back immediately, now recovering from her fall.

"Rubber gloves?" questioned Laurie.

"Protection from ectoplasm," Saskia retorted.

"Hand whisk?" asked Kennedy.

"It creates air currents." Saskia had an answer for

everything. Laurie picked up the last item: a big book. He read the title aloud. "*The Bumper Book of Scary Stories*. Does this help you come up with ideas when you're inventing your jobs?"

"What are you talking about?" Saskia stared at the three Squad members.

"You're more of a ghost creator than a ghost hunter, aren't you?" suggested Kennedy.

"You've somehow made this gladiator seem ghostly..." Laurie took a step closer to the suspected phantom faker.

"... and then you get paid to sort it out," finished Nabster.

"That's not true!" Saskia retorted hotly, her cheeks red. She was *really* annoyed at the accusation. "How dare y— wait! What was that?"

"Oh, here we go again." Kennedy folded her arms, unimpressed. "More humming, is it?"

"No... someone else spoke. Didn't you hear it?" Saskia stared around the empty room, the coil of plaits on top of her head quivering.

They all stood very still and very quiet.

Hicnoloesse.

"Who said that?" The ghost hunter was becoming more and more panicked.

"What?"

"Someone said..."

Hicnoloesse.

"It's coming from the gladiator!" Saskia pointed, her finger shaking with fright.

With that there was a **POP** and a puff of green

smoke floated out of the gladiator's helmet.

Hicnoloesse! repeated the voice as the smoke got

thicker. # AARRRGH!!!!

Saskia Spectre gave an ear-piercing shriek. "What's

that?! It really *is* a ghost!" she squealed, and clutched

her suitcase, consumed with fear.

"Don't you want

to catch a real ghost?"

asked Laurie, feeling a

little braver than the

last time he'd heard

the gladiator speak.

"You must be

joking!" cried Saskia.

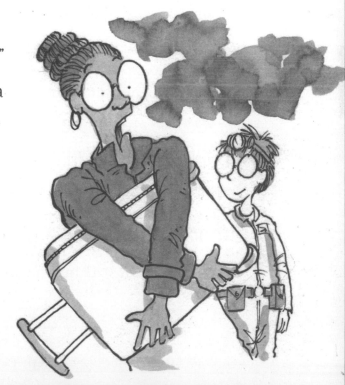

At this point three things became clear:

1. Saskia Spectre could run almost as fast as Kennedy.

2. The Musuem Mystery Squad were all a lot braver than she was.

3. Nabster had better equipment than any ghost hunter.

Grabbing his bag, Nabster quickly un-stoppered a sample bottle and swept it through the air, scooping up some of the smoke, before popping the top back on again. Half a second later he snatched his camera and began filming.

Kennedy slowly stepped towards the ghostly gladiator.

"Hello..." she said cautiously. "Can you hear me? Why are you here?"

Hicnoloesse! came the voice once more.

Then, just like last time, the smoke began to thin and

the armed fighter returned to being a normal museum exhibit once more. The ghost had come and gone.

Gus ran into the Roman Zone, having heard the commotion from the corridor, and witnessed Saskia Spectre's speedy departure.

"Did it happen again?" he asked.

"Yes, but this time I captured some smoke *and* filmed it!" Nabster raised a bottle and his camera proudly. "Now we have some real evidence to help us work out what's happening."

"What was up with our ghost-hunter friend?" asked Gus.

"At the first sign of something spooky, she was away!" said Laurie. "We can forget the idea that she created this ghost to earn some money – she was way too scared by it! I think we might have a genuine ghoul here!"

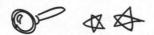

Kennedy's Diary

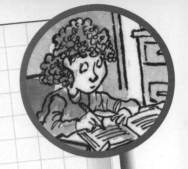

Thursday, 1.00 p.m.
Current UPDATE:
The Case of the Roman Riddle

- **Saskia Spectre:** probably still shaking, probably given up ghost hunting.
- **Magda Gaskar:** delighted not to have to pay Saskia Spectre's fees, but keen for answers to her gladiator problem.
- **Gus:** still tall, still not funny.
- **Laurie:** certain there is a real ghost.
- **Nabster:** certain there's not.
- **Gladiator:** now quiet, but we've heard it become quite chatty twice now.

Conclusions: Absolutely no idea what's going on. Arrrgh.

What next? Nabster collected smoke and recordings - let's see whether they tell us anything.

Sitting at the table in the HQ, Nabster's aqueduct trickled away above, but his mind was focused only on the gladiator samples he'd collected. He lined up his camera, voice recorder and the bottle of green smoke.

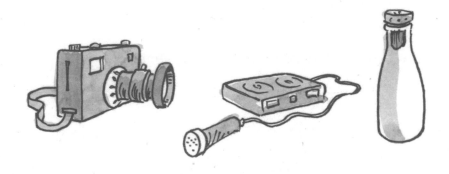

"Right," he said happily. "Evidence we can look at, listen to and smell!"

With a few taps on the keyboard, Nabster played the video footage he had captured, showing it on the laptop screen while they all watched. He slowed the action right down, moment by moment. The Squad saw Kennedy approach the gladiator, the smoke thin then disappear, and they even spotted Saskia Spectre speeding off like a frightened rabbit. It was good to see the day's events replayed, but it didn't really tell them anything new.

"What about the smoke?" Laurie reached over the table and pulled out the bottle's stopper a little, cautiously sniffing the contents. "A... a... aaa... tchoo!" He gave a violent sneeze and quickly shoved the stopper back in.

"Bless you," grinned Nabster. "You sound like Strickland. Atishoo... or whatever it was he said."

"In situ." Kennedy firmly reminded him of the Latin phrase.

"Hang on..." Laurie suddenly stopped rubbing his nose. "Kennedy, earlier you said that ancient Romans spoke Latin."

"Yep." Kennedy nodded, pausing.

"So, as a Roman, wouldn't the gladiator have spoken it too?"

Kennedy slapped her hand to her head. "Of course! You're right! The gladiator isn't talking nonsense. This Roman riddle is in Latin! We should be able to work out what it's saying!"

"What was the word again?" asked Laurie quickly.

"Hiccup lessons? Something like that..." Kennedy grabbed her diary to find her entry from earlier that day. "I wrote it down."

"Wait a sec. Here it is." Nabster quickly clicked on

the file from the voice recorder and played it at full volume through the wall screen's speakers: **Hicnoloesse!**

"Can you slow the sound, like you did with the video?" asked Laurie.

A few taps on the keyboard from Nabster and the voice slowed, stretched and deepened.

Hi-i-i-i-ck . . . n-o-l-o . . . ess-sse.

"Sounds like three different words," said Nabster.

"Could be," said Kennedy. "Time to learn some Latin."

Nabster's fingers were a blur on the laptop as he located a translation website.

"Try 'hick'," said Laurie. They watched the wall screen.

Q   hick   ✕

Q   hicc   ✕

Q   hic| ✕

Nabster nodded. "Yes, *hic* is a Latin word. It means 'this'."

"What about 'nolo'?" asked Kennedy.

Q   nolo| ✕

"Let me check..." Nabster examined the translation results. "Yes! It means 'I do not want'."

"And 'lessie'?"

Nabster typed in the final word.

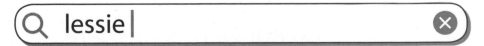

Q   lessie| ✕

"No, nothing there."

There was a moment of silent disappointment.

"What about 'essy' with a 'y'?" suggested Laurie.

| Q essy | |

Nabster checked, and shook his head. "No."

Laurie was about to retreat to his sleeping bag in defeat when Nabster cried, "Hang on! There's *esse*. Yeah, that's it. It means 'here'."

"Put the whole phrase in. *Hic nolo esse.*"

On the laptop screen, the words the gladiator had said over and over appeared for the Squad to see.

| Q **LATIN:** hic nolo esse | |
| **ENGLISH:** I do not want to be here |

The room fell silent.

It was Laurie who spoke first.

"That is *seriously* spooky! I told you it's a Roman ghost! That gladiator doesn't want to be stuck in a museum!"

"We've finally solved one part of the Roman riddle," said Kennedy. "We know what the voice is saying!"

"We have to work out *how* that exhibit is speaking." Nabster looked at his equipment spread out over the HQ table. "It *can't* be a ghost. I need more evidence to prove that. And I think I know how to get it."

WHO WOULD YOU RATHER FIGHT?

Gladiators were forced to fight some fierce opponents, including wild animals! Which of these ferocious beasts would you rather battle in the arena?

ELEPHANT (ELEPHANTIS)

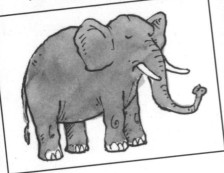

SPEED: 15 mph
STRENGTH: Largest land mammal in the world
WEAKNESS: Only land mammal that can't jump
RATING: ★★★

TIGER (PANTHERA TIGRIS)

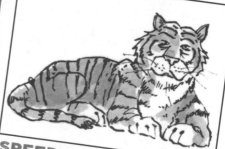

SPEED: up to 40 mph
STRENGTH: Teeth can be up to 10 cm long
WEAKNESS: Can't catch prey over long distances
RATING: ★★★★★

DID YOU KNOW...

It's thought that the thumbs-up signal came from gladiator battles. The emperor would make a thumbs-up or thumbs-down gesture to say whether a warrior would live or die!

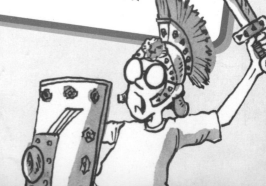

BEAR
(URSUS)

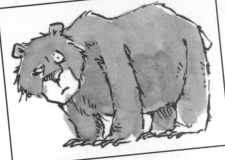

SPEED: up to 25 mph
STRENGTH: Front claws can measure up to 10 cm – as long as human fingers!
WEAKNESS: Hibernates for 6 months every year = sleepy!
RATING: ★★★★

CROCODILE
(CROCODILOS)

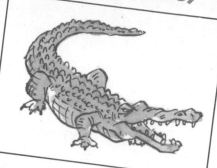

SPEED: up to 20 mph (in water)
STRENGTH: Strongest bite of any living animal
WEAKNESS: Slow on land
RATING: ★★★

COLIN
(COLINUS MAXIMUS)

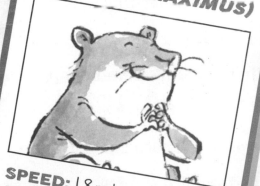

SPEED: 1.8 mph
STRENGTH: Can eat body weight in carrots
WEAKNESS: Too fond of carrots. Also very small
RATING: ★

DID YOU KNOW...

Some gladiators fought in the Colosseum – a huge amphitheatre that could seat 80,000 people. You can still visit the site today in Rome, Italy.

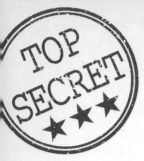

Chapter 8
In which there is a question about the cost of ghosts

All was peaceful in the Squad HQ. Nabster had run up to the Roman Zone to scan the gladiator now no one was there to complain about the ScanRay's humming. Kennedy was on her beanbag quietly writing and Laurie was completely still inside the safe cocoon of his sleeping bag (either snoozing or hiding from unhappy ghosts).

The only real activity was in the corner of the room where Colin the hamster had stopped sipping water and discovered a new game: pushing straw through the bars of his cage. He nudged a piece with his nose and watched it fall to the floor. Then he did the same again. He was having great fun. He hadn't worked out that he was slowly moving his comfy bed out of his own reach.

Kennedy glanced up as another piece of straw drifted downwards. "What are you doing, Colin? You're making a complete mess over there!" She turned her attention back to her diary, flicking through the last few entries. "I don't know if we'd have worked anything out yet if it hadn't been for Angus Strickland and his Latin sneeze!" she said.

"Oh yes, the man who values the treasure," recalled Laurie from inside his sleeping bag. "Do you know, he said it was good the helmet was bashed and cheaper, because it left more money to buy other things."

Kennedy looked thoughtful. "I know you think there's a *real* ghost, Laurie, but if Angus Strickland didn't want the museum to buy the helmet at all, then could he have invented a ghost to make sure the display went badly?"

Laurie's head popped out of his sleeping bag. "He said something about smaller objects being the real gems. Did you see the coins on his cufflinks? Maybe that's the sort of thing he wants the museum to buy."

"I saw him staring at the Roman coin collection before you spoke to him," said Kennedy.

At that moment the door burst open and a breathless Nabster rocketed into the room. Even Colin stopped his straw game to see what was going on.

"Wait till you see this!" Nabster propped himself up on the table to catch his breath. "Someone has definitely tampered with that helmet. There's all sorts of stuff in it that shouldn't be there!"

Laurie sat up sharply. "Like what?"

Nabster showed them the gladiator helmet's ScanRay results. "Proof that this headgear is not what it should be!" he said proudly.

The ScanRay screen showed a list of materials:

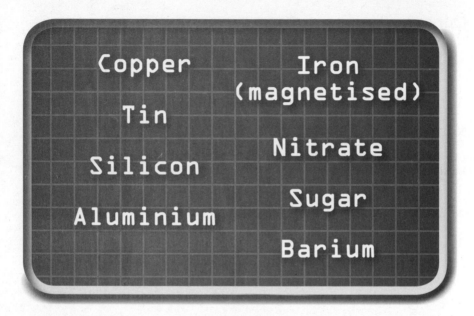

Copper

Tin

Silicon

Aluminium

Iron
(magnetised)

Nitrate

Sugar

Barium

"That seems quite a lot for a metal hat," said Kennedy.

"Well," said Nabster, "it's made of bronze – that's a mix

of copper and tin, but then look at all the other stuff."

"It's like a weird shopping list," said Kennedy.

"Aluminium? Sugar? Why?"

"If someone gave me a carrier bag with all of those things in it, I'd be making some microchips, and also—" said Nabster.

"Wait, what?" interrupted Kennedy. "We know the Romans were clever, but microchips are about two thousand years after their time!"

Nabster continued to explain (in wonderfully geeky detail) how these ingredients could be used to make wafer-thin microchips to power an electronic gadget, a tiny speaker and some exploding smoke pellets.

"And?" asked Laurie, still none the wiser.

"Don't you see?" said Nabster. "With either a timing device or a remote control, someone could set off a voice recording and a smoke bomb hidden inside the helmet."

"And create a ghost!" finished Kennedy with a grin.

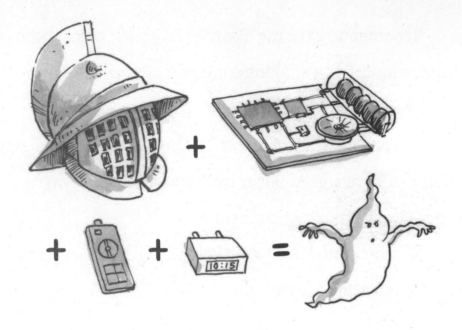

"Yeah, sorry Laurie," said Nabster. "I think our ghostly gladiator has been made up by someone very real."

"But who?" Laurie prompted.

"It would have to be someone who spent a lot of time alone with the helmet," Nabster suggested. "The device is too fiddly to set up while there are lots of museum visitors around. It would probably have been rigged before the helmet went on display."

"Before you arrived we were talking about how much time Angus Strickland must have spent assessing the value of the Taggart Treasure..." said Laurie.

"And we also wondered whether he might be happy to have a ghost story attached to the helmet, because he wants the museum to buy coins instead," added Kennedy.

"It's him! It must be!" Nabster agreed. "I have to admit, I'm pretty impressed by his gadget knowledge."

"But what's our next step?" Kennedy wondered aloud. "We can't just march up and accuse him of tampering with a two-thousand-year-old artefact. Somehow we have to catch him in the act."

Colin pushed another piece of straw through his cage and onto the floor. It was the first time Nabster had seen the mess.

"Oi, Colin! What are you doing? Look at the floor! You're making it look like a farmyard in here!"

"Hang on." Laurie was sitting up in his sleeping bag. "Farm... What do the folk who found the treasure trove on the farm think of the price Strickland has suggested for the helmet? Let's see whether we can find out."

A quick internet search located a recent news article from a West Lothian newspaper.

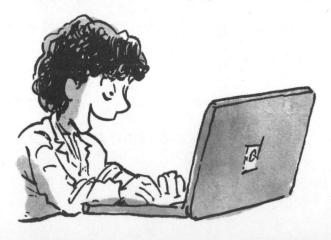

CHEAP TREASURE

TREASURE TROVE VALUATION CAUSES ANGER AT TAGGART FARM

Local farmer James Taggart was reported to be too angry to comment further today, after he called the valuation of the so-called Taggart Treasure "insulting". Treasure Trove specialist Angus Strickland said that damage caused by ploughing greatly reduced the value of a recently discovered gladiator helmet. Strickland's decision was described as final.

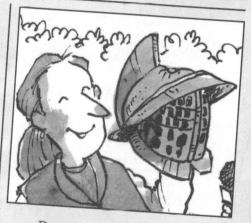

Despite this, the popular annual fireworks festival at Taggart Farm remains scheduled to take place next month.

"So Strickland *did* give a low value. We were right!" said Kennedy, as Nabster flicked through images of last year's fireworks at Taggart Farm. It seemed to be a big community occasion, and there were photos of crowds in a field below beautiful coloured sparks and a haze of red smoke.

"These pictures are giving me an idea," said Nabster. "What if we create our own smoky ghost? We could surprise Strickland with a taste of his own medicine!"

"I like that plan." Kennedy caught on quickly. "We'll watch his reaction to a ghost he's not expecting, and that will show us for sure that he's been controlling the ghostly gladiator!"

"But how do you make a ghost?" asked Laurie.

"Well, the ScanRay has just given me the list I need."

Nabster headed for his supply cupboards.

"I should have all of that stuff somewhere."

"First he doesn't believe in ghosts, and now he wants to *make* one," observed Laurie.

Colin sat back and nibbled on a carrot stick, having, in his own hamster-ish way, assisted the Squad in making a connection and coming up with a new plan.

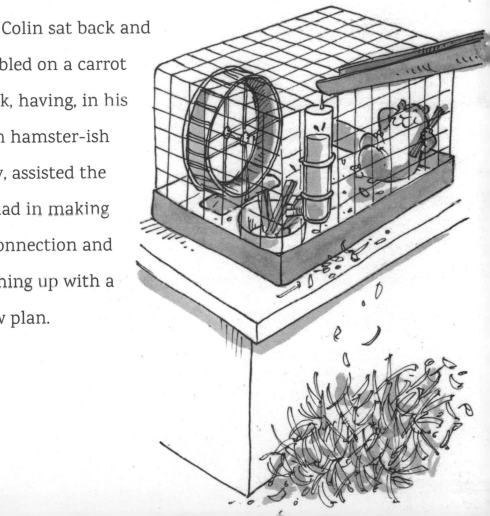

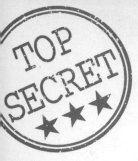

Chapter 9
In which a different Roman speaks

Nabster was looking as happy as Nabster could ever look. He was in his perfect world, a world in which he had worked out an ingenious solution to a technical challenge. He mixed and wrapped powders together and used his voice recorder to make a very loud, short message. Then, while he attached wires and switches to a Roman artefact he'd borrowed from the display, Kennedy called Gus on the walkie-talkie.

"Gus, can you meet us in the Roman Zone in one hour? Over."

"Yes, of course. What's up? Over."

"We believe a new ghost is going to appear. Over."

There was a long pause and some crackling on the line before Gus spoke.

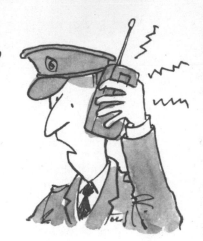

"What makes you think that? Over."

"Let's just say Nabster is working on it! Over and out."

Meanwhile, Laurie had dressed for the Roman Zone again. He tapped out an email to Magda marked URGENT.

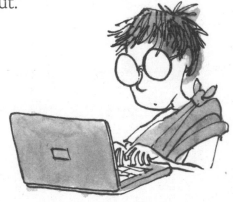

To: **Magda Gaskar, Museum Director**
Subject: URGENT Meet Roman Zone 1 hour

Dear Magda,

Our investigation of the Case of the Roman Riddle has reached a vital stage. We need you to come to the Roman Zone in one hour's time, and could you please bring Angus Strickland with you? There's something we'd like him to see.

Many thanks,

Museum Mystery Squad

Nabster grinned as he carefully put the last of his newly created equipment in his bag. Everything was set. A different Roman was about to come to life.

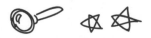

Nabster worked quickly and quietly in the Roman Zone, which had reopened to visitors. His preparation had been so skilful, he was ready in three minutes and no one had noticed what he was doing. He gave Kennedy and Laurie a nod and a thumbs-up.

A few visitors were pressing the buttons that lit up the lines of Hadrian's Wall and the Antonine Wall, while others peered at the motionless gladiator figure.

Gus arrived right on time, and gave the Squad a look that asked 'What are you lot up to?'

Magda and Strickland were hot on his heels. Magda glanced about nervously. Strickland did not seem at all pleased to be hustled back to the Roman Zone. His impatient voice carried around the room.

"Much as I find this area interesting, Magda, there are many other collections that need my attention."

With their prime suspect now in position, it was time for the Squad to act.

"OK," said Kennedy. "Let's do this."

"On it." Nabster hit a button on the remote in his pocket.

I HAVE A MESSAGE! boomed a loud voice.

Heads swivelled to see who had shouted.

I HAVE A MESSAGE! said the voice again. The gathered crowd realised it was coming from one side of the room and all eyes turned that way.

Suddenly, there was a sharp **POP** and red smoke seeped out from beneath a centurion figure's crested helmet. It clouded around the Roman soldier as the voice boomed out again.

I AM THE ONLY GHOST! I AM THE ONLY GHOST!

Shock from the visitors in the room turned to a buzz of conversation. Some fumbled for phones to film the extraordinary event. Gus threw a worried look at the Squad.

With Nabster's centurion ghost in full flow, the three Squad members turned their attention to Strickland.

He looked baffled. "Is this a new piece of art, Magda?"

"Er... I'm not exactly sure." Magda turned to Nabster, Kennedy and Laurie for an explanation.

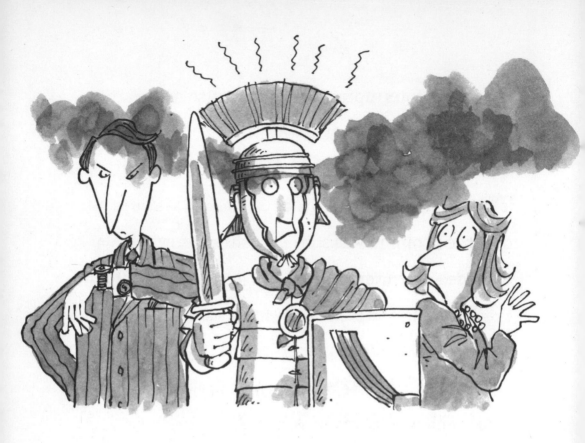

"Strickland doesn't seem that bothered!" whispered Kennedy out of the corner of her mouth.

Laurie was puzzled. "Why isn't he reacting?"

"I thought my ghost would surprise him!" said a very disappointed Nabster. "I don't understand—"

He was interrupted by a disturbance at the entrance to the Roman Zone.

"What's going on here?!" It was Jimmy, Gus's new joking friend. He had dropped his takeaway coffee all over the floor and was staring in disbelief at the smoke-shrouded centurion.

Before anyone could answer, the centurion figure's booming voice filled the room again:

I AM THE ONLY GHOST! I AM THE ONLY GHOST!

Jimmy moved towards the figure in a daze. "Why is *that* one speaking? And why is the smoke *red*?" He pulled a small remote control out of his coat pocket and shook it, as if to make sure it was working.

All eyes were on him.

He looked up sharply, realising what he'd done.

"What's that you've got there, Jimmy?" Gus asked suspiciously.

"None of your business," snapped the man. "And it's James, not Jimmy, if you don't mind!"

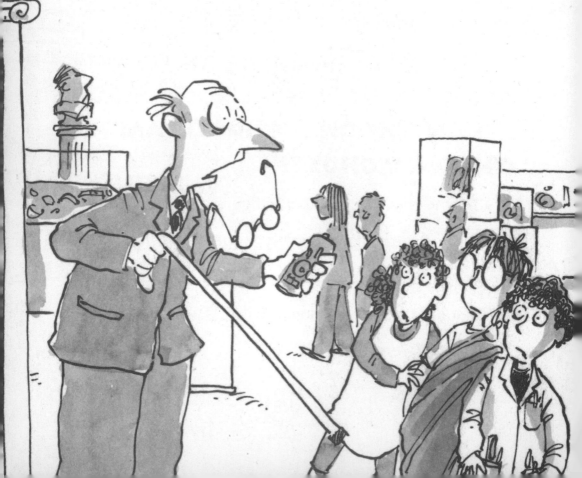

"James…" repeated Kennedy. She'd heard that name before in this investigation. "James… James Taggart… You're not *farmer* James Taggart, are you?"

"Yes, I am," said the man crossly. "And that gladiator helmet is mine!"

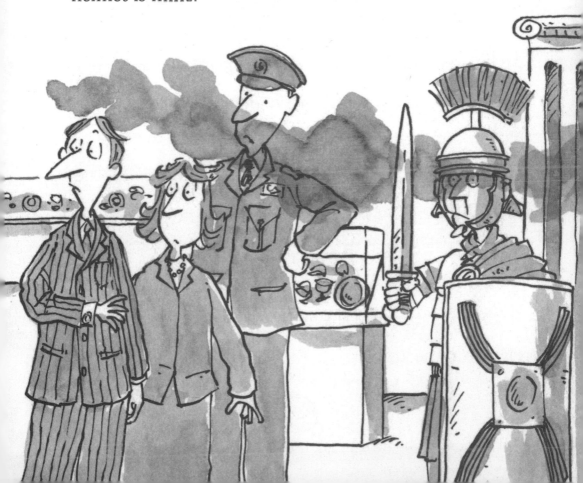

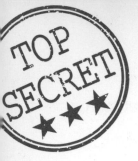

Chapter 10
In which marble columns
are inspirational

All friendliness and joking had now disappeared from

James Taggart's eyes, and he no longer seemed so

elderly and frail. Throwing his walking stick to the

ground and straightening himself to his full height, the

farmer threw a steely glare at the Squad and took off

at speed. He dodged through the throng of bewildered

museum visitors, swerved round the stuffed tiger and,

reaching up, grabbed the ancient helmet from the

gladiator's head.

But in his haste he accidentally set off the remote control in his pocket.

Hicnoloesse! The Latin voice began. With a **POP** green smoke began to emerge from the helmet Taggart was clutching under his arm. He sped towards the exit.

There was chaos in the room now. Red smoke. Green smoke. Ghostly voices coming from two different places, echoing off the pillars.

Hicnoloesse!

I AM THE ONLY GHOST!

Taggart ran, with Gus chasing after him. There was so much smoke the farmer began to disappear.

"He's behind the marble columns!" shouted Kennedy.

129

With that, Nabster was reminded of
something he'd thrown into his bag when

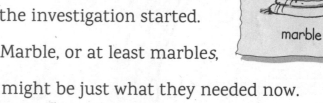

marble

the investigation started.

Marble, or at least marble**s**,

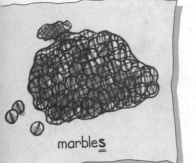

marble**s̲**

might be just what they needed now.

He hurled the bag of marbles

through the air across the Zone. It

burst open on the tiled floor just in front of Taggart,

scattering glass balls beneath his feet. The escaping

farmer lurched unsteadily, waving his arms for balance

as if slipping on ice.

Spotting her chance, Kennedy ran to the now

bareheaded gladiator and grabbed the net from its hand.

With a mighty effort she launched it as hard and as

high as she could.

130

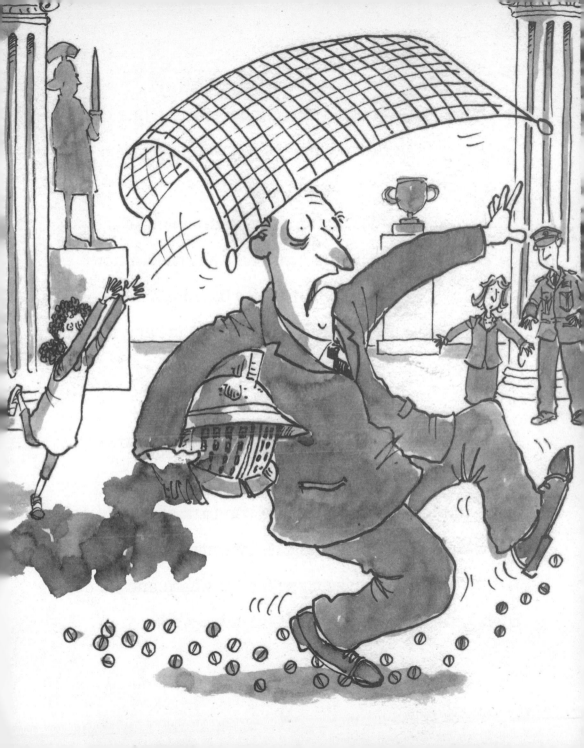

It landed on top of the skidding man, bringing him down with a crash. He collapsed, cursing, in a tangled heap.

Gus moved in and reached under the net to retrieve the stolen gladiator helmet. It had picked up a new dent in Taggart's crashing fall. Spotting this, Strickland commented loudly, "I'm afraid you've knocked a few more pounds off the value of that exhibit, Mr Taggart."

"You! You've already under-priced it!" screeched the outraged farmer. "I want this helmet back! Private collectors will give me thousands more than you!"

"Can someone please explain what exactly is going on here?" demanded a bewildered Magda Gaskar.

"This is James Taggart, the farmer who ploughed up the Taggart Treasure," explained Kennedy.

"He was trying to turn the treasure into a problem for the museum," said Nabster. "If he could make everyone think the helmet was haunted, he figured the museum wouldn't buy it."

"Then he would get it back," finished Laurie.

"That land has been in my family for centuries," cried the farmer, still trying to fight his way out of the gladiator's net. "Whatever I dig up should be mine! I shouldn't have to give it away for some stupid tiny amount!"

Nabster picked up the remote control that Taggart had dropped in the chaos. "I'm guessing years of organising fireworks festivals meant that you knew all about timers and explosions," he said. "Once you knew the valuation, you agreed to bring the helmet to the museum, but you'd placed these gadgets inside it. You could set off smoke capsules and voice recordings from wherever you were sitting in the Roman Zone. And some you timed to go off overnight or to scare the cleaners in the morning."

Taggart scowled. Nabster was clearly spot on.

Gus looked stony-faced at the man he had thought of as Joking Jimmy. "Right," he said. "I don't think you'll be laughing at much of what I say next. We're off to the police station."

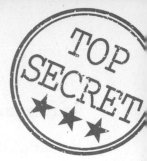

Last chapter
In which the case is closed

A week later and the ghostly voices and smokebombs

of the gladiator and the centurion were slowly fading

into memory. All was back to normal in the Museum

Mystery Squad HQ. Laurie had tidied away his toga and

jumpsuit. Kennedy had written up a full report of the

Squad's findings. And the HQ's leaky pipe had finally

been fixed, which meant there was no longer any need

for Nabster's aqueduct. He was disappointed at having to

dismantle such a triumph of engineering, and cheered

himself up by putting the marbles used to catch James

Taggart in a jar as a memento from the Case of the Roman Riddle.

The Squad had received a very grateful email from Magda earlier that day. Not only was she delighted that the case had been solved and the cleaners were back at work, she noted that there had been a surge in visitor numbers. It seemed people wanted to see the 'ghostly gladiator' for themselves – although the figure was now an ordinary museum exhibit.

"It says in the news that the museum will definitely buy the Taggart Treasure," reported Nabster as he skimmed an article on his laptop, "and that James Taggart *will* get money for it!"

"Really? After all he did?" asked Laurie from inside his sleeping bag.

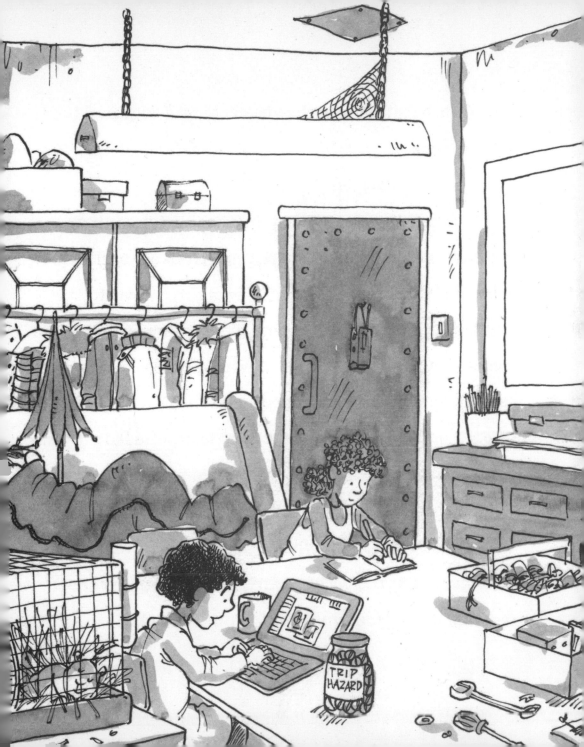

"Yeah, but it also says he's been charged with fraud, and he'll have to pay the museum's costs for dealing with the so-called ghost."

"If there's any extra money, maybe the museum can buy some new coins. I'm sure Angus Strickland would love that!" Kennedy grinned.

Nabster got up from the desk to fill Colin's water feeder (he had to do it himself now that the leaky ceiling and the aqueduct were gone). "I'm glad Colin has stopped making a mess," he said, and fed the Squad's furriest member a carrot. "Even if he did helpfully remind us to think about the farm."

"That straw got everywhere," said Laurie. "I even found a piece at the bottom of my sleeping bag."

"How did it get down there?" Kennedy laughed.

"Well it wasn't me. But I have thought of another possibility." Laurie wriggled his eyebrows mysteriously behind his glasses.

"What's that?" asked Nabster.

"A Stage 2 poltergeist moving things around, of course. Perhaps there's a ghost in the museum after all..."

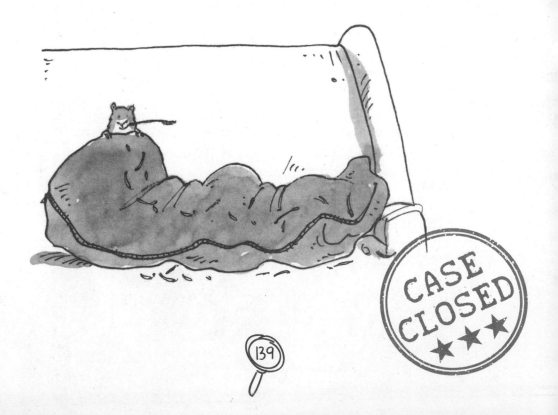

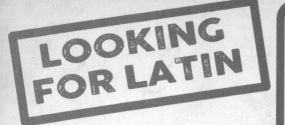

LOOKING FOR LATIN

There are lots of words we still use today that came from Roman times. Can you help the Squad find all of the Latin words in this wordsearch?

ALIBI   ULTRA   BONUS

VICE VERSA   TERROR   AQUA

ET CETERA   ALIAS   AUDIO

ABACUS   IN SITU   DICTATOR

EXIT   POST   VICTOR

SINISTER

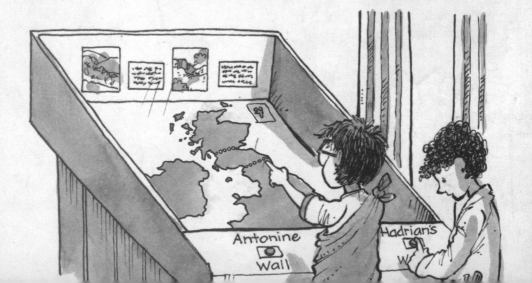

Antonine Wall

Hadrian's W

A	U	L	T	O	R	E	B	H	E
X	D	E	R	A	Q	U	A	U	C
B	I	M	G	S	A	U	D	I	O
H	C	A	R	T	L	U	R	N	I
A	T	C	A	B	O	N	U	S	T
L	A	B	A	C	U	S	X	I	V
E	T	E	R	O	R	R	E	T	I
S	O	A	B	A	T	A	P	U	C
O	R	L	B	O	I	U	S	O	E
V	C	I	E	A	X	D	I	B	V
I	M	B	O	L	E	A	G	A	E
C	S	I	N	I	S	T	E	R	R
T	B	L	U	A	G	E	S	L	S
O	A	L	I	S	S	V	I	O	A
R	E	T	C	E	T	E	R	A	P

Answers at the back

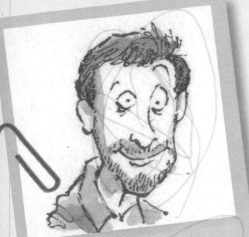

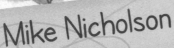
Mike Nicholson

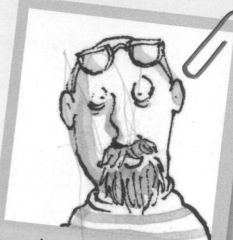
Mike Phillips

Mike Nicholson is a bike rider, shortbread baker, bad juggler and ear wiggler, and author of the *Museum Mystery Squad* series among other books for children.

Mike Phillips learnt to draw by copying characters from his favourite comics. Now he spends his days drawing astronauts, pirates, crocodiles and other cool things.

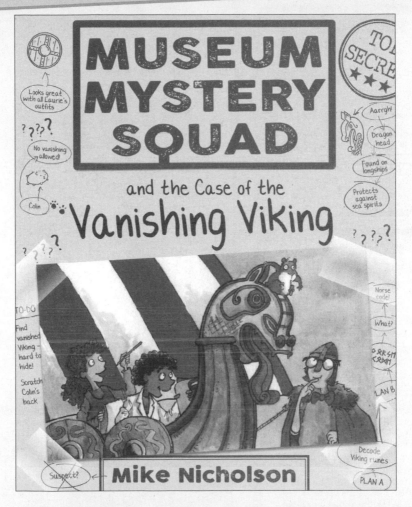

A Viking has vanished from the
museum's longship: can the Squad
solve the mystery, or will they
be left all at sea?

ANSWERS

LOOKING FOR LATIN
(Page 140)

A	U	L	T	O	R	E	B	H	E
X	D	E	R	A	Q	U	A	U	C
B	I	M	G	S	A	U	D	I	O
H	C	A	R	T	L	U	R	N	I
A	T	C	A	B	O	N	U	S	T
L	A	B	A	C	U	S	X	I	V
E	T	E	R	O	R	R	E	T	I
S	O	A	B	A	T	A	P	U	C
O	R	L	B	O	I	U	S	O	E
V	C	I	E	A	X	D	I	B	V
I	M	B	O	L	E	A	G	A	E
C	S	I	N	I	S	T	E	R	R
T	B	L	U	A	G	E	S	L	S
O	A	L	I	S	S	V	I	O	A
R	E	T	C	E	T	E	R	A	P

DATE DECODING
(Page 22)

LV	=	55 B.C.
MLXVI	=	1066
MDLXXXVII	=	1587
MDCCCXXXVII	=	1837
MCMXVII	=	1918
MCMLXIX	=	1969
MMIII	=	2012

ROMAN INVENTIONS
(Page 52)

STRAIGHT ROADS: Romans built their roads as straight as possible so their armies could move as fast as possible. Winding roads take longer to travel and could hide bandits.

NEWSPAPERS: Roman newspapers were written on metal or stone.

TOILETS: Roman toilets were flushed with water from aqueducts! (Like Nabster's aqueduct only much bigger and not made of Lego...)

CALENDAR: The 'Julian' calendar was named after the Roman emperor Julius Caesar.

BOOKS: Books are made from paper, and paper is made from tree trunks.

THE SCANRAY: No! The ScanRay is not a Roman invention, it's a Nabster creation!

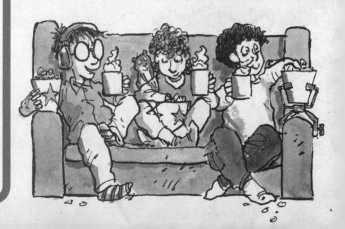